Living with AIDS and HIV

WITHDRAWN

This book is dedicated to all those who
are living, and have lived, with AIDS and HIV

Living with AIDS and HIV

David Miller

Principal Clinical Psychologist and
Honorary Lecturer in Psychiatry and
Genito-Urinary Medicine
The Middlesex Hospital Medical School
London

with a guest chapter from
Chris Carne

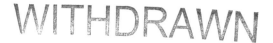

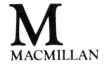

MACMILLAN

First published 1987
Reprinted 1987, 1988, 1991

Published by
THE MACMILLAN PRESS LTD
Houndmills, Basingstoke, Hampshire RG21 2XS
and London
Companies and representatives
throughout the world

Distributed in North America by
SHERIDAN HOUSE PUBLISHERS
145 Palisade Street, Dobbs Ferry, NY 10522

Typeset by Footnote Graphics, Frome, Somerset

Printed in Hong Kong

British Library Cataloguing in Publication Data
Miller, David, *1955-*
Living with AIDS and HIV.
1. AIDS (Disease)—Psychological aspects
I. Title
362.1'969792   RC607.A26
ISBN 0–333–43243–6
ISBN 0–333–43244–4 Pbk

Contents

Acknowledgements

I am especially proud to acknowledge the enormous help and support of many persons in the development of this work. For the past two and a half years, I have been a co-facilitator of a fortnightly group for people with AIDS, their families and loved ones, run under the auspices of the Terrence Higgins Trust. This is really the group's book, for they have provided the inspiration and ideas for much of what is written here. We have certainly learnt a great deal together. Other people with HIV, PGL and ARC, members of Body Positive, and my patients, have made as great a contribution to this work. Their courage, honesty, insight and humour have been a constant inspiration in these past four years. They have offered the most enriching examples of human striving and the most valuable lessons in every sphere of personal and professional practice. To them all, I offer my deepest thanks. I am indebted to Roger Osborne, formerly Senior Editor, The Macmillan Press, for his readiness to offer support and encouragement in the face of much delay; and I offer my grateful thanks also to Chris Carne, Ian Weller, John Gallwey, George Leach, Don Jeffries, Tony Pinching, Riva Miller, Alana McCreaner and Jane Miller for their stimulating ideas, their exemplary modelling of the best standards of clinical practice, their helpful suggestions regarding manuscript changes, and their support. The problems discussed have been ours. They are presented here in the hope that they will be of help to others who have had to, and will, face the enormous challenge of living with AIDS and HIV.

Introduction

THE NEED FOR THIS BOOK

AIDS is, at the time of writing, still the subject of considerable misunderstanding and fear, both in those who may be infected with the causative virus, HIV (Human Immunodeficiency Virus)*, and in those who care for people infected and with disease. This misunderstanding persists for some good reasons. First, the popular media have been slow to develop a responsible stance in reporting the infection (it is still common to see persons infected with HIV being equated with people with AIDS). Second, the infection and disease is still widely regarded as a 'gay' disease, and stereotyping of patient groups and prejudice against lifestyles held to be responsible for the passage of HIV into the general community have stood in the way of greater social under-standing and acceptance of those at risk. Third, HIV and AIDS are new. This means that people generally are not yet sufficiently aware of the disease and its presentation to become familiar with it. This appears to be the case particularly in the health professions, especially in areas away from the major medical teaching centres, where AIDS patients are more common and treatment regimens are more practised. To have HIV or AIDS is, in many places, to be a medical novelty. In some instances, this means being a 'guinea-pig' in the formation of particular medical policies and practices.

The newness of the infection and its disease states does not mean that the disease is not understood. Since AIDS was first reported in the medical press in mid-1981, it has become possibly the most intensively researched medical phenomenon ever, with many governments allocating millions of pounds world-wide to help further our understanding of both the disease and its cause. Much indeed is now understood about the virus. In particular, the ways in which it is transmitted are well and reliably understood. This means that we know how to stop the virus spreading.

As the range of medical and social knowledge about the virus grows, it is clear that this knowledge must be passed on as widely as possible.

*Previously known as HTLV-III or LAV (see Chapter 1).

HIV is not something to fear—it is something to fight. But to fight it effectively, everyone affected—patients, (para)medical staff, and carers (lovers, spouses, families, friends, work colleagues)—must be clear about what this phenomenon means on a social, medical, practical and emotional level. And they must learn to communicate this knowledge effectively. For so many of my patients, fears aroused by their diagnosis or knowledge of infection have been matched by their fears about the reactions of those around them. It is most important that our management of this infection and its diseases be not clouded by intolerance, prejudice or fear. AIDS is a disease, and HIV is an infection, in which all 'victims' are innocent.

AIMS OF THIS BOOK

As a counsellor who has worked with many hundreds of people with HIV and AIDS for the past four years or so, I have been surprised at some of the difficulties involved in establishing resources available for counselling those affected in parts of the United Kingdom away from the London area. While working at St. Mary's Hospital in Paddington, my colleagues and I founded the first comprehensive workshops in Great Britain for medical and health staff working with patients. These have been particularly successful in educating many staff about the infection and its diseases. However, not all those infected will seek or wish to be counselled by doctors and their colleagues, and not all health staff have the required knowledge. For many, personal knowledge of infection and/or disease will be a lonely and confused battle, characterised by despair and fear. They will not know to whom they should or could safely turn. Many have been confused by differing approaches to particular issues related to their health. For example, while some patients have reported that their plans for a controlled health-food diet have been encouraged by their doctors, others have said their physicians have dismissed such initiatives as 'a ridiculous waste of money and effort'. Who is right? Many patients have asked 'Who do I believe?' when confronted by choices about the 'best' drug regimen, or even the 'best' safer sex advice.

The aim of this book is to help in making choices easier for patients and their carers when facing such confusions. It is not, as such, a medical textbook. Rather, it is intended as a practical guide to coping with the problems raised by HIV. The range of chapter subjects reflects the issues most frequently raised in my experience with AIDS-related counselling. If the book could be summarised in a couple of phrases, they would be: 'Keep communicating', 'Master the facts to master your circumstances' and 'Have courage and a sense of history'.

1

The Virus and Its Spread

THE VIRUS

The agent responsible for AIDS—Human Immunodeficiency Virus (HIV)—is a *retrovirus*. This means that it belongs to a family of viruses that have a unique ability—they make DNA (the 'blueprint' for genetic replication) out of RNA. 'Ordinary' viruses do not do this: with them the process of viral replication occurs the other way round— DNA produces RNA. Because this unique family works the opposite way, i.e. backwards, they are called *retro*viruses.

Retroviruses are a very complex family of viruses that were first isolated and characterised from animals in 1970. Examples of animal retroviruses that have been found since that time include the feline leukaemia virus, which causes an AIDS-like range of infections (more often than it does leukaemia) in cats; the African Swine Fever Virus (ASFV), which in pigs causes AIDS-like immunological abnormalities and some of the symptoms seen in humans with AIDS; the Visna virus, which affects sheep; and the bovine leukaemia virus—an infection in cattle. Perhaps the closest animal retrovirus relative to the AIDS virus in humans is the Simian T-cell Lymphotropic Virus-III (STLV-III), which has been responsible for diseases in monkeys. This virus originates from the African green and macaque monkeys, and comes up again in discussion later.

It wasn't until the late 1970s that members of the retrovirus family were found to infect human beings as well. Until the subsequent isolation of the AIDS retrovirus, which was then called Human T-Lymphotropic Virus III (HTLV-III) by the Americans, and Lymphadenopathy-associated Virus (LAV) by the French (and is now known universally as Human Immunodeficiency Virus—HIV), there were just two known human retroviruses.

The first, Human T-Cell Leukaemia Virus (HTLV-I), causes leukaemia, and is passed from mothers to children in the womb, between adults through sexual intercourse, and through blood transfusions. It, like many other retroviruses, is a 'slow' virus—it can take 40 years or more to express itself as disease in the infected host. The other interesting feature of HTLV-I is that only 1 in 100 of those infected actually develop disease—the other 99 appear to be simply carriers. The second relative in this strange human family is HTLV-II, which seems to be transmitted in the same way as HTLV-I, but as yet shows no evidence that it is actually associated with a disease. It was originally isolated from two patients with 'hairy cell' leukaemia, but does not appear to cause this disease itself—its isolation was a 'chance finding' in these patients. If HTLV-II does cause a disease, it has yet to be found. Both of these retroviruses appear to be spreading slowly in the population, but there is no evidence to indicate that they are causing widespread disease.

It was due to these two prior discoveries in man that the retrovirus causing AIDS could be isolated. If the AIDS epidemic had occurred ten years earlier, the technology available to isolate the cause would have been inadequate. What the laboratory techniques now available can tell us is that the three members of the HTLV family are all distant cousins—there are no very close resemblances across them, and they do not cause the same diseases.

Much more recently, a fourth member joined the family. It was originally called HTLV-IV, or LAV2 (depending which side of the Atlantic one was working), although it is now known by the internationally agreed name of HIV2 (Human Immunodeficiency Virus 2), and was first isolated from West African prostitutes by French scientists. It differs significantly from HIV, but despite hopeful first reports suggesting that it might be less pathogenic (i.e. leading to less severe disease), it also causes AIDS. It is known to be different from the original AIDS virus because the antibody tests which isolate HIV antibody only pick up HIV2 50 per cent of the time. The virologists who made this discovery suggest that this later virus evolved independently from HIV, and that it is more similar to STLV-III than to HIV.

The story of the discovery of HIV is interesting in itself[*]. When the epidemic of AIDS hit San Francisco and New York in 1981, there was intense speculation about why previously rare skin cancers and opportunistic infections were affecting a basically healthy population of young men. As other groups became tragically involved, such as injecting drug users and haemophiliacs, it was becoming clear that the cause of this devastation was a transmissible agent—the appearance of the illness in haemophiliacs who were using blood-clotting agents from donated blood testified to that. But what was it? Many possible agents

[*]The story of the race to discover the cause of AIDS is explained in *AIDS: The Story of a Disease*, by J. Green and D. Miller (Grafton Books, London, 1986).

were scrutinised as possible causes, including cytomegalovirus (CMV), Epstein–Barr virus (EBV), hepatitis B virus (HBV) and ASFV. The problem was that, while some or all of these viruses were found in some people with AIDS, many patients did not show signs of infection by them.

The pace quickened when it was discovered that an AIDS-like disease appeared in cats infected with the feline leukaemia virus. While this virus cannot be passed on to humans, attention focused on the possibility that a retrovirus might be the cause of human AIDS. In 1983 a study at Harvard in the United States showed that 40 per cent of AIDS patients tested had antibodies to HTLV-I. This suggested that if a human retrovirus was responsible, its antibodies might be 'cross-reacting' with the HTLV-I antibody test. The antibodies showing up on the tests used in the study related to the envelope of the known HTLV viruses—a promising sign. At around the same time, in mid-1983, a team of researchers from the Institut Pasteur in Paris, led by Dr Luc Montagnier, announced that they had isolated a new retrovirus from a male homosexual with Persistent Generalised Lymphadenopathy (PGL) (which was, at that time, thought to be suggestive of the inevitable onset of AIDS). This new virus was distinct from the other known human retroviruses, and was named LAV—Lymph-adenopathy-associated Virus. Confirmation that this was indeed what researchers had been looking for came shortly after from America, where Dr Robert Gallo announced that a new retrovirus had been isolated from people with AIDS in a number of different centres—the problem was that they could not be compared, as they could not be 'grown' in sufficient numbers, and transmission of the virus to other cells could not be reproduced. Therefore, it could not be determined whether they were in fact different isolates of the same virus or indeed whether this was the virus causing AIDS.

The final breakthrough in the struggle to characterise the agent responsible for AIDS came when the American team developed a permissive cell line, thus enabling the new virus to be cultured and cross-matched. They called it Human T-Lymphotropic Virus III (HTLV-III). Once the ability to grow the new intruder and test its activity in the laboratory had been mastered, blood from many patients was tested and the news that the cause of AIDS had been found was confirmed.

HIV has the following structural properties.

1. It has an envelope—an outer membrane about two millionths of an inch in thickness. This envelope is very vulnerable to destruction by heat, detergents and organic solvents such as alcohol.

2. Inside the envelope there is a 'core' of proteins and genes—the genome. The three major genes are the 'gag' gene, which makes the specific core proteins the virus contains; the 'env' gene, which makes the envelope of the virus; and the 'pol' gene, which makes the vital chemical reverse transcriptase—the element that makes it possible for the virus to manufacture DNA from RNA. A vital fourth component is called the transactivator or 'tat' gene, which appears to regulate replication of the virus (a major research effort is being conducted to find ways of turning the 'tat' gene off, so that the virus no longer replicates in the body). This collection of genes is best imagined as a ruler, with centimetres marking off the different genes. At both ends of the ruler are pieces called 'long terminal repeats' or LTRs. Their function is to help slot the virus into the genome of the cell that the HIV is invading, and to switch it on.

3. It is now widely considered that the structure of the virus may change as it is being transmitted from one person to another. These changes are slight but significant—they may account, for instance, for the variations in the HIV isolates found in Africa, England, France and the United States. Isolates from Africa show far more variability than those found in the West, possibly because they have had a longer time to evolve. More intriguing still is the recent discovery that, while it remains in the infected host over a period of time, the virus appears to mutate on its own. The full significance of this discovery has yet to be assessed. The greatest variation overall appears to be in the envelope genes.

4. The closest structural relative of HIV is the Simian T-cell Lymphotropic Virus found in the African green monkey. It seems possible that HIV has done something that other retroviruses have done very rarely—it has crossed from animals to man. Just quite how this has occurred is unknown (although some bizarre speculation about possible routes certainly has resulted).

5. The main destructive effect of HIV occurs through its selective attacking and destruction of specific immune cells in the blood and tissues—in particular, a subset of lymphocytes or cells known as T_4 lymphocytes. It is thought that the genes in the central area of the genome are actually involved in the expression of disease. The process of T cell infection by HIV is shown in Figure 1.1. As the diagram shows, the first step involves the virus (called an 'antigen' because the body recognises it as a foreign 'invader') becoming attached by areas of its envelope to a receptor on the surface of the T_4 lymphocyte. Normally, as other 'conventional' viruses appear in the bloodstream, they are

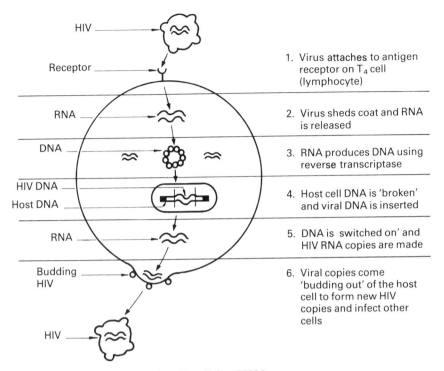

HIV

Receptor

RNA

DNA

HIV DNA
Host DNA

RNA

Budding
HIV

HIV

1. Virus **attaches** to antigen receptor on T_4 cell (lymphocyte)

2. Virus sheds coat and RNA is released

3. RNA produces DNA using reverse transcriptase

4. Host cell DNA is 'broken' and viral DNA is inserted

5. DNA is switched on' and HIV RNA copies are made

6. Viral copies come 'budding out' of the host cell to form new HIV copies and infect other cells

Figure 1.1 Infection of a T cell by HIV

picked up by antigen-presenting cells, whose job is to show the foreigner to B cells and other immune cells, one of which will carry a special chemical (an 'antibody') which sticks to the antigen's surface. Once this has occurred, B cells start replicating at a quick rate, thus reproducing more antibody, which, in turn, attracts other cells, which engulf and destroy the invading virus and all copies of it in the bloodstream and elsewhere. Other chemicals, amplifiers of immune response such as interleukin-2 and gamma-interferon, are also produced by T_4s to assist in viral destruction. However, for some reason this does not occur to the same degree with HIV or HIV2. Part of the reason lies in the extraordinary ability of HIV to attract antibodies mainly to those parts of its structure that are not crucial for maintaining reproduction—it can thus continue attacking cells and replicating while undergoing antibody attack. Also, the virus may be constantly changing the nature of its envelope, making it more difficult for it to be identified and attacked.

The process by which HIV enters the lymphocyte via the receptor (also called the 'T_4 antigen') involves bits of the HIV being 'studded' on the outside wall of the lymphocyte. Released antibodies appear to attach to these particles and kill the cell in which the virus is located. The most favoured target for HIV is those T cells (T lymphocytes) which produce chemicals called 'lymphokines'. Lymphokines help B cells to recognise antigens (foreign bodies) and to start antibody production. As such, they are frequently known as 'T-helper' cells; those that are not infected or invaded by HIV also appear to be made less effective. The net result is that the body's antibody production and efficiency is dramatically reduced. As if that were not enough, other T cells (cytotoxic or 'cell-killing' T cells—also known as 'T-killer' cells), which can normally attack cells infected by viral invaders without antibody assistance (they destroy the viral invader's cell membrane), also seem to be rendered less effective, even though they are not themselves directly infected. The overall result is that a depletion of helper cells, and the reduction of killer cells, leaves the body prey to all sorts of infections which could normally be easily fought off.

Once inside the target lymphocyte, the HIV sheds its coat and produces an extraordinary chemical, an enzyme called reverse transcriptase; thus, from a single strand of RNA a double strand of DNA—a copy of the virus—is built. The next step in infection and replication then takes place. The DNA strand in the host cell or lymphocyte is broken, and the HIV DNA is inserted. Once inserted, the inserted virus cannot be distinguished from its host. The restructured DNA is 'switched on', although this may be after a long 'dormant' period—perhaps lasting many years—and copies of HIV are created. There is still much speculation about what causes or 'triggers' this reproductive process; some researchers think that it may occur when the T lymphocyte responds to the presence of other antigens by reproducing itself—thus, more copies of the virus are also made. However, the presence of the 'tat' gene within the HIV genome enables the HIV component of the host to reproduce itself very much faster than the host lymphocyte can (some say possibly up to 1000 times faster).

The final stage of the viral reproductive cycle involves the viral copies 'budding' out of the host lymphocyte and moving off to infect other T-helper lymphocytes, thus adding to the immune destruction in the body. In the process of replication and budding off, the host T-helper lymphocyte is itself eventually destroyed; once a certain number of these cells have been destroyed, the body cannot restore its required supply of vital antibody-stimulating T-helper lymphocytes, and AIDS (Acquired Immune Deficiency Syndrome), with its devastating range of infections and tumours, is the result.

It should be understood that the virus attacks that part of the immune system known as the 'adaptive immune system'. There is much more to the immune system than this part only, but it is the vital part and is thus critical for the maintenance of health in the face of opportunistic infections.

EPIDEMIOLOGY

There seems to be little doubt that the HIV epidemic originated in Africa, although this is still often vigorously refuted by some African governments, who regard the virus as having been brought to Africa by 'promiscuous' North American tourists. The main evidence for an African origin is that the closest known relative of AIDS-creating viruses is STLV-III, found in the African green and macaque monkeys. It seems pretty likely that HIV and HIV2 have somehow crossed over to humans, as discussed above. Studies of stored African blood indicate that HIV has been around for perhaps 10–15 years or even longer, so in general terms it cannot be called an old virus which has only recently manifested itself in disease.

The spread of HIV from rural Africa probably coincided with the migration of people from rural to developing urban areas. The late 1960s and 1970s have been times of considerable economic change in many African states, not least with broadening tourist industries. In many parts, middle-class city life is associated with relatively high numbers of sexual partners, young men, in particular, visiting prostitutes on a regular basis while away from their rurally located wives and families. It is clear that high proportions of female prostitutes in some African cities have HIV infection, and the prevalence of infection in many countries in Africa is already frighteningly high. In this context of an established sex industry and increasing tourism, it is easy to imagine the potential for HIV infection spreading to many other countries.

For a while it was considered that Haiti was a source of HIV infection in the United States—low incomes and high levels of poverty resulted in a sub-industry of male prostitution catering for American tourists there. However, contrary to earlier speculations, it seems most likely that from Africa the virus gained a foothold in America, and it was then exported to Haiti by American tourists. The rising seroprevalence in Europe has reflected initially the broad patterns of colonial links between some European and African countries (e.g. France and Belgium).

One fact that has been clear to many researchers working on the African experience for some years is that the epidemiology of the epidemic in Africa shows clearly that HIV is spread through heterosexual sex, from male to female and *just as easily* from female to male. This crucial fact is only now being taken seriously in the West, where in many places the HIV pandemic (a world-wide epidemic) is still regarded (and perilously trivialised and dismissed) as a 'gay plague'.

Routes of Transmission

Since mid-1981 when the epidemic was in its relative infancy, two of the major risk groups for future HIV infection have all but disappeared from the epidemiological map—haemophiliacs and recipients of blood transfusions. However, back in 1981–1982, as the roll of casualties tragically unwound, the major risk groups included:

Homosexual and bisexual men.
Haemophiliacs and recipients of blood transfusions.
Needle-injecting drug users.
Haitians.
Sexual partners of persons in these groups.

Current experience has shown that the common factors uniting these persons were sexual intercourse and/or blood-sharing (including exposure to blood and/or blood products). Of course, we now know that HIV-infected semen, blood and vaginal/cervical secretions are the three richest sources of potential infection to other persons, and these were the fatal links in the development of the world-wide AIDS tragedy. (The full range of bodily fluids that have been associated with the AIDS virus, and their level of known infectivity, are discussed in Chapter 4.) Knowing this, and realising that the infective agent was a transmissible virus, enabled some infection-control steps to be taken in those countries where widespread disease was occurring, so that now all blood being donated for medical use is screened for antibodies to HIV. Where this infection is found in donated blood, it is retested to ensure that a mistake has not been made. If it is still positive, the donor of that blood is recalled to the donation facility, and another sample is taken and double-tested. If this again proves 'positive', the donor is informed and asked to refrain from future blood or body-product donation, and the blood is destroyed. A similar process occurs with donations of semen and other bodily fluids, ensuring that people receiving such donations receive a gift that is free from infection. By this means, haemophiliacs, blood transfusion recipients, organ recipients and women attempting pregnancy by A.I.D. (Artificial Insemination by Donor) are no longer at risk for infection through infected body-product donations.

The remaining major risk groups for HIV infection really depend on the numbers of persons in the general population with the infection.

For example, it is clear from many studies that HIV is not a disease affecting simply gay men and injecting drug users *and* that it is spread from men to women and women to men. Therefore, it is most realistic and prudent to classify *risk activities* and not risk groups. This is not to deny that in the West, at least, gay men and injecting drug users are at most risk if behaviour changes to reduce their risk are not adopted on an individual basis—in some countries these populations already have high levels of infection and so more cases of AIDS-related illness can, sadly, be expected to appear in the future. However, we now know enough about the way HIV is spread to be able to say that in all societies avoidance of infection can be assured provided that there is no bodily fluid exchange during sex; no sharing of needles and other equipment that may be contaminated with (possibly infected) blood; and no pregnancy in those women already infected. These are the three remaining risk areas. Detailed information on safer sex and risk-reduction is presented in Chapter 4.

THE ANTIBODY TEST

The HIV antibody test is actually an Enzyme-Linked Immunosorbent Assay (ELISA). In the United Kingdom a version of this—the Competitive ELISA—is used as the first test, and a different technique, the Western Blot, is then used in blood-screening laboratories as a confirmatory test if the ELISA indicates the presence of antibody. The antibody test is specific to HIV antibodies—it will not show the presence of antibodies to other infections such as herpes, for example. What happens is this: Blood from the patient is placed into 'competition', to bind with antigen in a small 'well', with a human HIV antiserum which has been coupled with an enzyme. Additives—a substrate—are included in the mix. If HIV antibody is present in the patient's blood, there is no conversion of the added substrate to its coloured end product—a clear mixture indicates that the blood is infected. If there is no infection, however, the mixture colours.

A positive result arising from this procedure can be considered very accurate. The percentage of inaccurate results is surprisingly low for a test that was developed with new materials 'from scratch'. False-positive results (i.e. results indicating that the fluid sample is infected with HIV when in fact it isn't) occur in 0.25 per cent of 'true negatives'—i.e. in 25 out of 10 000 cases. False-negative results, however, may occur in up to 4 per cent (4 out of 100) cases of 'true positives'. It was for this reason that persons who suspected themselves of being at risk for infection were asked to refrain from donating blood at blood transfusion centres and mobile blood-donation facilities; if they continued to do so, there was a slight risk that infected blood could still get into blood banks. Another difficulty with the testing process is that persons exposed to the virus may take some months before evidence of their having been infected is detectable. In most cases seroconversion occurs within twelve weeks of exposure (if it is going to occur at all). In a minority of cases seroconversion may take up to twelve months (longer in a very few cases). Therefore, if a person has not yet seroconverted after exposure to HIV, the test will not show it and he or she will be deemed seronegative.

The problems with false positives and false negatives may be a thing of the past soon, as more accurate tests are currently being developed. For the time being, it is fair to say that if a person's behaviour indicates that he or she may have been at high risk of exposure in the recent past, his or her blood will be very carefully tested to ensure that any such errors are absolutely minimised.

For any person contemplating having the HIV antibody test, it is important to consider just what the test can tell us and what it can't. The test *is not a test for AIDS*. The test does not give a diagnosis, in the way that one receives a diagnosis of a disease. It simply provides a laboratory-derived marker that one has been infected by a specific virus. As such, it is a mistake to say 'I've been diagnosed seropositive' if you are seropositive; better and more accurate to say you've been '*found*' or '*identified*' seropositive.

The test provides no other information. For instance, if HIV antibodies are identified in your blood, it does not tell how long you have been infected, how severely infected you are, how infectious you are to others (although for safety's sake you are presumed constantly infectious for life, or at least until an effective antiviral agent is found and administered), or whether you are going to develop disease in the future or not. It is this relative lack of information that has led many social groups to suggest that where potential pregnancy is not a factor in consideration, little will be gained from having the antibody test except considerable and often unremitting anxiety, as identified seropositives simply 'wait for the worst to happen'.

People contemplating having the test done should be very clear about their reasons for doing so. Most will want simply to know whether they are seropositive, perhaps after having experienced high-risk sexual activity in the past. For them, however, the important question is this: 'What extra use will this information be to me—how is it going to help?' For people from groups with a known high prevalence of infection, it may be reasonable to assume that they have been exposed to the infection in the past and that in order to ensure that they do not pass it on or acquire further infection(s) in the future, they should consider adopting safer sex and other risk-reduction practices at all times from now on. Having a positive test result will certainly not assist this process by itself. It can't help diagnostically in identifying disease (and HIV-related disease is well identified medically without the need for antibody screening in almost all cases).

Being identified as seropositive will also carry burdens other than the emotional. Numerous practical consequences arise, including being barred from taking up endowment mortgage policies and medical insurance; many dentists and even some medical doctors may decline to offer treatment; and many employers who may learn of a person's seropositivity will terminate his or her employment or decline employment to prospective employees. Each of these circumstances can have a major (usually detrimental) effect on the way a person lives.

Some people may wish to have the antibody test for other reasons: for example, they may have had sexual intercourse with a person whom they later suspect to be at risk for this infection. This becomes a worry when they consider the consequences for starting a family or starting future sexual relationships. Some people may have felt unwell for a time, or have minor illnesses that are persistent or not easily explained—having the antibody test will be a means of eliminating HIV as a possible cause. In other cases, people may have required blood transfusions at the time when the cause of AIDS was unknown, and they have been worried since that they may have been infected in this way. Whatever the reasons for wishing to have the test done, the considerations discussed above apply just as fully. For this reason, *no one should have the antibody test without pre-counselling by an appropriately experienced counsellor.* HIV counsellors can be contacted at most sexually transmitted disease clinics, or via your doctor or community agencies concerned with AIDS and HIV.

2

The Clinical Manifestations of HIV Infection

by
Dr Chris Carne

Lecturer in Genito-urinary Medicine,
The Middlesex Hospital Medical School

The majority of HIV seropositive people feel entirely fit and well either all the time or most of the time. Any physical symptoms which a seropositive person experiences are most likely to be due to conditions entirely unrelated to HIV. After all, being infected with HIV does not make one immune to other diseases. Neither does HIV make one more prone to common infections such as colds or flu, so a cold which is slow to clear up should not be taken as a sign that the immune system is impaired.

The acquisition of HIV most commonly takes place during sexual intercourse or, in the case of intravenous drug users, when sharing needles or syringes. This is followed by the development of antibodies to HIV. In most cases these are detectable on the anti-HIV test within 3 months of acquiring the virus, but in a very few cases the development of detectable antibody may take as long as 12 months or possibly even longer. This process of developing antibody is known as 'seroconversion'.

Some people feel ill at the time they seroconvert, but more frequently there are no symptoms at all at this time. Why these differences exist is a mystery. If an illness occurs, this is most likely to take a form similar to glandular fever. In this event fever is accompanied by generalised swelling of the lymph glands, aching of muscles and joints, a sore throat and sometimes a rash. This usually lasts 3–14 days and is known as an 'acute retroviral illness'. These symptoms are very similar to those caused by classical glandular fever (infectious mononucleosis), which is a much more common disease. Very rarely HIV may affect the nervous system at this stage. This nervous system involvement may take the form of meningitis,

13

resulting in severe headache, fever and an inability of the eyes to tolerate light. Any illness that occurs at the time of acquiring HIV is self-limiting. It will get better in a matter of weeks, and no treatment is required other than simple measures such as analgesics for headaches, and rest.

PERSISTENT GENERALISED LYMPHADENOPATHY

When people have been infected with HIV for months or years, they may develop a generalised swelling of the lymph glands, especially at the back of the neck or in the armpits. This condition is known as persistent generalised lymphadenopathy (or PGL). The condition has quite a strict definition—i.e. glands must be greater then 1 centimetre in diameter in two different areas of the body for at least three months, and swollen glands in the groin do not count. Most other antibody positive people also have some degree of swelling of their lymph glands for a variable period of time.

Glands will tend to fluctuate in size. They tend to swell if the body is being stressed in any way—for instance, by getting overtired or contracting another infection. They are also inclined to ache at these times. Neither glandular swelling nor aching should give cause for concern, since they represent the affected person's way of fighting the virus. But aching or increased swelling should be taken as indications to take things easily. Over the course of a few years there is a tendency for the glands to gradually decrease in size. Again this is an entirely natural course of events. Only when glands have been swollen for a long time and then suddenly disappear is there any cause for concern. Similarly, if the glands suddenly swell up in one area only, it is worth consulting a doctor in case this is caused by a separate problem.

Antibody positive people with or without lymphadenopathy are prone to certain common skin conditions. Commonest among these is seborrhoeic dermatitis, which causes redness and scaling in the area of the eyebrows and moustache, and in the folds on either side of the nose, as well as on the trunk and limbs. Other common conditions to occur in anti-HIV positive people are folliculitis (an infection of the hair follicles), xeroderma (dry skin), bacterial and fungal skin infections and shingles (a painful reactivation of the chickenpox virus causing a rash on the face or trunk which is virtually always confined to one side of the body). People who suffer from genital herpes often find that this becomes more troublesome when they are antibody positive.

Some symptoms that may occur in antibody positive people are an indication that the immune system is somewhat impaired, although they do not warrant the term AIDS. Such symptoms include fever or diarrhoea persisting for more than a month for no cause other than HIV, and loss of more than 10 per cent of body weight. Another ailment that implies some immune suppression is when thrush causes white flecks or soreness of the gums. People with these types of symptoms are sometimes referred to as having ARC (AIDS-related complex). People with these symptoms are unwell as a result of their HIV infection and are more prone to progress to AIDS than others who are anti-HIV positive and well.

One symptom often experienced by people with HIV diseases such as PGL and AIDS is periods of fatigue, which may be very severe and which may appear without warning. These episodes may last for days or weeks, and their severity can vary greatly.

AIDS

AIDS affects only a small proportion of HIV-infected people. Several studies have shown that about 10 per cent of people progress to AIDS within three years of follow-up. However, the average incubation period of AIDS is over five years, so the proportion of people who progress is bound to be higher than 10 per cent over longer follow-up periods. Once someone is infected with HIV, the virus will almost certainly remain in the body for life. AIDS and HIV have not been recognised for long enough for us to understand the full natural history of the infection, so it is not possible to say what proportion of infected people will ultimately develop AIDS.

People with AIDS may suffer either life-threatening opportunistic infections, or tumours, or both. The term 'opportunistic' implies that the causative organism is completely harmless except to the immunocompromised. The life-threatening opportunistic infections fall into three main categories: those affecting the lungs, those affecting the gut and those affecting the nervous system.

Approximately half of all people with AIDS have a respiratory infection as their first sign of AIDS. Although there are several different organisms which can cause lung problems in AIDS, by far the commonest is *Pneumocystis carinii*, which causes pneumonia. This is an organism which is present in the lungs of many people and does no harm unless they become immunosuppressed. Normally it is present in very small numbers, but in an immunodeficient person it takes the opportunity to multiply and thereby causes pneumonia. Most of the common infections suffered by people with AIDS come about in this way: by reactivation of an organism that has been in the body a long time rather than from organisms that have been recently acquired.

Pneumocystis carinii pneumonia (PCP) presents with a dry cough, breathlessness and fever. The symptoms tend to gradually get worse over the course of several weeks. The diagnosis is usually suggested on the chest X-ray, which frequently shows a diffuse hazy shadowing quite unlike other pneumonias. It is treated with high doses of an antibiotic called Septrin (cotrimoxazole), usually given intravenously into an arm vein. Sometimes a different drug called pentamidine is used. The large majority of AIDS patients suffering from this form of pneumonia will recover when treated in hospital but they are at risk of getting a recurrence. For this reason, patients may then be asked to take a low dose (a so-called maintenance dose) of Septrin or a similar drug, to try to prevent recurrences.

Opportunistic infections affecting the gut may take various forms. First, 'thrush' (also known as candidiasis, from the causative organism—*Candida albicans*) may affect the gullet, causing discomfort on swallowing. This falls under the definition of AIDS as opposed to thrush in the mouth, which is not so serious. These conditions usually respond very well to antifungal drugs which can be taken by mouth, but sometimes thrush in the gullet requires a drug which can only be given intravenously. Various infections may cause diarrhoea, the commonest of which is caused by an organism called *Cryptosporidium*; this can be very resistant to treatment. Quite frequently, when AIDS patients suffer from diarrhoea, no opportunistic organism can be found, and in this situation the mainstays of treatment are simple antidiarrhoea drugs, of which there are many to choose from. Another common gut manifestation of AIDS is severe ulceration of the anal area by genital herpes. Fortunately, the drug Acyclovir is extremely effective in combating this condition.

The nervous system may also be affected in a variety of ways. Some of the neurological disorders seen in AIDS patients are not opportunistic infections or tumours but, rather, are the primary neurological effects of HIV. The commonest of these disorders is called subacute encephalitis, which causes a gradual loss of intellectual function which may progress to severe dementia. HIV may also sometimes affect the spinal cord or peripheral nerves, causing weakness of the legs and abnormalities of sensation. A fungus called *Cryptococcus* may cause meningitis (i.e. an inflammation of the membranes that cover the brain and spinal cord). This results in persistent headache and fever, and what is known as photophobia (an abnormal visual intolerance to light). The condition requires hospital treatment with intravenous drugs, and this is usually followed by maintenance therapy with an antifungal drug. Other patients may suffer from cerebral toxoplasmosis, which can cause fitting, headache, drowsiness and weakness of a limb or limbs. The diagnosis is made by a sophisticated kind of X-ray technique called computerised tomography (CT or CAT scan), and treatment is by a combination of drugs (often sulphadiazine, pyrimethamine and folinic acid). A virus called cytomegalovirus (or CMV) may inflame the retina of one or both eyes, causing a condition known as CMV retinitis. This causes impairment of vision, which if left untreated can progress to blindness. Fortunately, the recently developed drug DHPG (or Gancyclovir) is of considerable benefit in combating this complication.

By far the commonest tumour to affect AIDS patients is a form of skin cancer called Kaposi's Sarcoma (KS). This tumour was very rare before the advent of the AIDS epidemic, but it had been seen in the so-called classical type in elderly men of Mediterranean descent, in central Africa (different from the AIDS KS seen there) and in some people on immunosuppressive drugs. These various forms of KS differ somewhat in their appearance and behaviour.

The form of KS seen in AIDS patients is almost always more aggressive than the other types. It usually starts on the skin, but, unlike the classical type, it can start anywhere on the skin surface. In the very early stages it appears as a small pink or purplish patch on the skin, often measuring a few millimetres in diameter. Commonly there is a bruise-like brownish yellow stain around new lesions (i.e. spots) of KS. These lesions are painless and non-itchy. If one runs a finger over a lesion, it feels like a thin disc rather than being just a stain on the surface. KS very rarely goes away spontaneously. With time, lesions may increase in size, appear elsewhere on the skin surface and spread to internal organs.

Occasionally KS starts in other organs such as a lymph node. In others it may start in the gastrointestinal tract, in which case the first lesion may be seen on the palate. Lesions in the gut may bleed and thus cause anaemia. Spread can occur to any organ in the body, brain and lung involvement being particularly serious.

The aim of treating Kaposi's Sarcoma is to improve the quality of life and hopefully to prolong it. At present it is not realistic to expect to cure the condition entirely. Treatments may be classified as local or systemic (i.e. general). Local treatments are mainly used for cosmetic purposes—for instance, for lesions on the face or other exposed parts of the body. One commonly used approach is local radiotherapy. The dose of rays used is very small and the beam is directed only at the lesion to be treated, so that no damage is done to other tissues and none of the side-effects associated with high-dose radiotherapy arise. Sometimes KS may obstruct the drainage of fluid from certain areas of the body such as the feet, causing oedema (i.e. swelling due to enlargement of the tissues with fluid). Radiotherapy can be used to reduce the swelling and can also be helpful if KS lesions become painful. Other local treatments that can be used are surgical excision of lesions or injection of cytotoxic (anticancer) drugs into the lesion.

Systemic treatments are of two main types: cytotoxic drugs or alpha-interferon.

The term 'cytotoxic' implies that the drugs kill cells, and can thus cause regression of KS lesions. However, their effect is not specific for cancer cells, so they tend to kill other cells in the body and, if used in high doses, they can cause serious side-effects. These unwanted effects depend on which drug or drugs are used, but, in general, there is a risk of killing rapidly dividing cells such as blood cells, some of which are important to the functioning of the immune system. For this reason a balance must be struck between the beneficial and the adverse effects of these drugs. When they are used, the dose employed is low, in order to minimise side-effects, and often a combination of different drugs is used.

Alpha-interferon is a protein which forms part of the body's immune system. It can now be manufactured and has been used experimentally in a variety of different illnesses. Recently it has been licensed for use in the UK against Kaposi's Sarcoma. It has both immune-stimulating and antiviral effects, and is given by injection several times a week. Roughly speaking, about one-third of patients treated with interferon show improvement, about one-third stay the same and about one-third continue to deteriorate. Unfortunately, even in those patients who show improvement the effect is only temporary (often lasting about a year), although some people get a much more prolonged response. Interferon tends to make people feel unwell, with flu-like symptoms, so, in order to minimise this, a small dose is given at first and then gradually increased. Fortunately, this adverse reaction to the drug decreases as treatment progresses.

A far less common tumour in AIDS patients is non-Hodgkin's lymphoma, which is a cancer of the lymphatic tissue—i.e. the type of tissue found in lymph glands, which is also present elsewhere in the body. This tumour is common in non-AIDS patients, but falls within the definition of AIDS if it starts in the brain or if the patient is anti-HIV positive. Non-Hodgkin's lymphoma is treated with cytotoxic drugs, but among AIDS patients the response to treatment is poor.

Many different paths are being followed by research workers in their attempts to develop an effective treatment for AIDS. Several of the drugs which have reached the stage of clinical trials fall into the group known as reverse transcriptase inhibitors. Reverse transcriptase is an enzyme—that is, a kind of protein—which enables the genetic information carried by the virus to be transferred into DNA, which carries genetic information in human cells (see Chapter 1).

Reverse transcriptase is vital to the spread of the virus within the body. By inhibiting this enzyme, it should be possible to prevent the

Table 2.1 Classification of HIV infection

Group I   Acute infection (glandular fever-like +/− meningitis)
Group II   Asymptomatic infection
Group III   Persistent generalised lymphadenopathy
Group IV   Other disease

    A. Constitutional disease (fever)>1 month/diarrhoea>1 month/ weight loss > 10%)
    B. Neurological disease (dementia/HIV disease of spinal cord or peripheral nerves)
    C. Secondary infectious diseases
       1. Life-threatening opportunistic infections—e.g. PCP
       2. Non-life-threatening opportunistic infections—e.g. oral candidiasis
    D. Secondary cancers (Kaposi's Sarcoma/Ab+ve non-Hodgkin's lymphoma/primary lymphoma of brain)
    E. Other conditions (other symptoms, infections or cancers that may be associated)

Categories C1 and D are classified as AIDS

---

virus spreading to infect more cells in the immune system. Drugs that fall into this group include HPA-23, Suramin, Foscarnet and AZT. Antiviral drugs, if effective, should be able to prevent further damage occurring to the immune system.

Another group of drugs, known as immune modulators, may be used to stimulate the immune system. These include drugs such as gamma-interferon, interleukin-2 and isoprinosine. If used alone, there is a danger that they may encourage the virus to multiply. So it is possible that the best treatment will be a combination of an antiviral drug and an immune modulator.

In the few years since AIDS was first recognised, diagnostic procedures have improved, allowing some conditions to be diagnosed sooner and thus improving the prognosis. Doctors have also become more knowledgeable about how best to use the existing drugs, and new drugs have been developed such as DHPG, which is very useful in the treatment of complications caused by cytomegalovirus. The use of low doses of antibiotics as maintenance therapy has been successful in delaying or preventing relapses of PCP. Much is still being learnt about the management of the various complications of AIDS, and treatment is steadily improving.

3
Coming to Terms with Diagnosis and Being Seropositive

When I was first diagnosed, I needed information and fast—there just wasn't anything available. I was 'stranded'.

When I was diagnosed, I was completely ignorant and I thought I would be dead within weeks. Nobody told me otherwise.

On diagnosis I had a great yearning for knowledge. Apart from depressing medically oriented literature there was nothing available.

The diagnosis came as a shock, but it was a relief to know what the cause of my long-term illness was.

With the shock of the diagnosis there came a sort of paralysis of the mind. It is absolutely *vital* that there is a swift follow-up in the days after so that a patient's many fears and questions can be [addressed and] answered.

When I first discovered that I was antibody positive I felt shock and disorientation. I woke up in the mornings shaking, had problems sleeping, and lost my appetite. I wrote a will, drank heavily, and seriously considered suicide. I thought, like others, that I was bound to develop AIDS.

I just couldn't believe it.

These statements are from people with AIDS and people who are seropositive. They all mention that hearing the news of their condition was a cause of considerable shock, and most mention that their greatest need at this time was for *information*. Experience suggests that the information should concern (a) the infection or disease itself, and (b) what to do about it. But first, some notes about shock.

SHOCK

People in a state of shock typically report feeling confused and bewildered. The mind seems to be in a constant turmoil, perhaps flitting from one thing to another, without reference to what is happening 'outside'. In this state it is almost impossible effectively to assemble a list of priorities, to concentrate, or to remember things clearly. Many people who have asked precise questions about their diagnosis or antibody result at the time they have been told will ask them again later, having forgotten that they ever asked the questions in the first instance, and the replies that followed.

Some people will become very emotional when the news is broken. They may start crying and 'breaking down', or they may be more aggressive, using abusive language and even physical aggression. Other people may respond by becoming quiet, withdrawn and uncommunicative. They may appear to have 'switched off', making it difficult for loved ones and staff to show that they care and are there to help. Whatever the person's reaction, it is important to remember that he or she is facing a life-threatening issue. No matter how reassuring the doctor, how promising the future for drug therapies, how minimal the physical impact of the infection, or how prepared intellectually the person may have been, news of infection or disease will be seen as having 'life or death' significance. No one can predict just how he or she might react to such news (despite any preparation). Members of 'high-risk' groups may well understand that their risk of exposure to HIV is considerably greater than that faced by others in the population, but if they have not yet been tested or become ill, they will probably still have had hopes for being free of HIV. News of infection or disease will therefore dash any such hopes, and the struggle they may have observed many times in others will suddenly become theirs, too.

Shock is a misleading and confusing state also for those caring for seropositives and patients. This is because the way shock reactions appear can be so unpredictable. Some people appear to manage the news very well at the time they are told, giving no particular signs of outward distress; they may then 'break down' a day or two later, once the impact and significance of the news have sunk in. When loved ones start behaving 'strangely' or out of character, perhaps by becoming aggressive or by losing all patience, it can be difficult to know how to react. There is the fear of adding to the patient's distress by becoming too assertive or returning anger. Some lovers and spouses have said that they 'seem to be doing everything wrong' at such times. Further problems arise when people who are told that they have AIDS 'block off' the news, and appear to act as if nothing is particularly wrong. Some people manage to do this for many months, only to face the full

Table 3.1   Some common shock reactions to diagnosis or infection

Emotional

Numbness/'stunned' silence/disbelief

Confusion/distractability/uncertainty—about the present and future circumstances

Denial ('It can't be true'; 'Don't worry, things will be fine')

Despair ('Oh my God, everything is ruined')

Anger—towards health staff, loved ones, etc., over impact on life and circumstances

Fear—of pain, death, disability, loss of bodily/mental functioning, loss of confidentiality/privacy

Guilt/self-recrimination—over the association of infection or illness with sexual activity, or with being gay or a drug abuser

Acute and severe anxiety (see Chapter 5)

Emotional lability—moving quickly and unpredictably from tears to laughter (and vice versa)

Sadness and morbid concern—for the future, work, lover/spouse/family, health

Suspicion—over the actions and behaviour of staff/loved ones/helpers

Relief—at knowing what the cause of recent illness is

Behavioural

Crying—episodic and often unpredictable

Anger and irritability—towards anybody, often 'sparked off' by trivial and important events (may be physical and/or verbal)

Withdrawal—distancing from the present issues and circumstances; reluctance to become involved in conversation, activities or plans for treatment

Self-denigration—referring to self as being 'deserving of this plague', worthless, 'unclean and dirty'

Impulsiveness—acting without thought for consequences

Bodily checking—for 'signs' of further infection or physical deterioration

Questioning—for reassurance, further information

impact of the trauma of diagnosis when they have become ill and too weak to keep their defences up. At such times, carers will be in the position of 'reliving' the time of diagnosis, only they are doing it this time *with* the patient, instead of alone.

It is important to remember that shock reactions, whatever their nature, are *a normal response to life-threatening news*. Remember, no matter what the news is, it will usually be seen as catastrophic, because of the popular (though often inaccurate) association of HIV or AIDS with death. Many writers have described how responses to a diagnosis of AIDS or news of HIV infection often mirror the reactions of patients being told that they have cancer and other serious illnesses. As such, the shock of diagnosis may persist for many months, or simply a few days—it is difficult to tell.

For loved ones and carers of people receiving such news, the question most often asked is: 'What can I do to make things better or easier?' This brings us back to the need for *information*—that which most of our patient statements have clearly described as being the most important need at the time of diagnosis or antibody result-giving.

INFORMATION

It has been clear from discussions with many patients that they have been so shocked by their news that they could not remember or think clearly for some time; therefore any information they were given at that time was not fully appreciated or 'taken on board'. However, many other people expecting to be told that they were seropositive, or that they had AIDS, have said that insufficient information was offered to them at the time their expectations were confirmed. Some have said that their questions were not answered at such times, or that the staff giving them the news 'seemed in such a hurry that I didn't want to bother them'. Others have complained that questions have been answered in medical language that they did not understand. As a result, they have gone home or remained in their hospital bed in a state of distress and with unanswered fears haunting them as they tried to come to terms with the situation. Of course, time is usually in very short supply in hospital clinics or wards, and it is not always possible for doctors or other staff to spend more than a few minutes with their patients. However, patients deserve, and indeed have the right to, reasonable time from health staff so that the diagnosis or antibody result can be discussed and put in perspective. It is, after all, a matter of life and death for many. Where there is a spouse, lover, family member or friend who is aware of the immediate circumstances, he or she may help enormously at this time by asking questions on behalf of the person involved. The staff's ethical requirements will require that they always ensure that the carer has the confidence of the patient—that he or she is bona fide. They can do this simply by asking the patient before they answer any questions. Importantly, in order to get useful information, it is helpful to *prepare questions in advance*, so that time is saved and the desired information is received.

Some health staff may find it difficult to discuss the significance of a diagnosis—perhaps they are unused to managing or discussing serious illness (especially when it is the patient who is asking the questions). Others simply may not know the full story, and are reluctant to discuss things they are not sure of (remember, at the time of writing there is still a great deal left unknown about AIDS and HIV). However, problems can arise when, perhaps in the quest for a sense of authority in difficult circumstances, the staff respond to questions such as 'How long have I got to live?' with a definitive statement such as 'Eighteen months— perhaps two years'. Such a statement can be and has been made even when the doctor has not been asked. The problem is, of course, that the staff have no way of knowing the truth of such a statement; they may well be quite wrong, and in the meantime they may have contributed to a sense of hopelessness and depression in a person who most needs a sense of hope. The best medical response to such questions (with unknown answers) is to say 'I (we) don't know. However, this is what we do know . . .'. The issue of prognoses, and other important issues, are discussed more fully below.

As for other things that carers can do at the time of diagnosis or result-giving, it is useful to remember that the patient will have many worries as a result of the news. Such worries (see Chapter 5) will add greatly to the patient's burden. Encouraging the patient to talk about or 'ventilate' concerns, worries or fears may be especially helpful, as they may concern questions for which there are simple or straightforward answers. There may be some initial reluctance from people to do this. They may, for example, attempt to protect the loved one from their own anxieties (and vice versa)—on the premise that a burden shared is a burden doubled. Or they may simply be afraid of the answer. Whatever the reason, we have found as a general rule that information helps, and communication helps. Other patients have said that at the time shortly after diagnosis what they most needed was human contact and touch. Holding hands, having a hug, just being there with them may be the most important help that carers (including hospital staff) can provide. Making such gentle contact also provides a good *model* for those who may be unsure about whether it is safe to do so. It helps to emphasise that this is not an infection to fear—it is an infection to *fight*.

Similarly, do not be afraid to show that you care and feel concerned, whether by displays of emotion or by practical organisation. The important thing is to be aware of the patient's tolerance for such displays (the issue of relationship adjustments is discussed in Chapter 6).

INTERPRETING THE DIAGNOSIS OR ANTIBODY RESULT

What does it mean to have AIDS or to be antibody positive?*The exact medical issues are discussed fully in Chapter 2. In this chapter we are concerned more with the ways in which such news is understood or interpreted by the patient.

For people who have been told that they are seropositive, it is crucial to remember that this is *not* the same as having PGL, ARC or AIDS. Being seropositive means that one has been exposed to the virus and has become infected as a result. A person in this state may be described as a 'carrier', although he or she is presumed to be infectious to others through the reliably understood routes of particular sexual activities, blood, blood and body products, and pregnancy. Thus, being seropositive for HIV means that one has an *infection*, not a disease or illness. As such, a positive antibody result is not a diagnosis, in the sense of a diagnosed disease or illness. The antibody test simply provides a laboratory-derived description of infection (see Chapter 1).

On the other hand, PGL, chronic HIV infection (what used to be known as ARC) and AIDS, while all being different clinical conditions, *are* diagnoses, as they all involve states of clinical disease or illness from the relatively benign state of PGL, to the more clinically serious state of chronic HIV infection, and then AIDS. If you have been told that you have PGL, chronic HIV infection or AIDS, then you have received a diagnosis according to the clinical signs described in Chapter 2.

Whatever the nature of the medical news you have received, it will often come as a great shock. The shock may be worse if there has been no previous hint of illness or HIV infection, or if there was no indication that blood was being actually screened for antibodies. Experience with many people in this situation suggests that, aside from the shock and desire for information mentioned by the patients in the opening section, many people will 'automatically' assume from then on that they are going to die. Some people have even said that despite having little or no outward sign of illness, they feel that their illness or infection must be obvious to others, as though they were wearing it like a badge. They have then withdrawn from the world, taking on a role of the 'terminally ill' patient, speaking and behaving in a way that seems to reinforce their (often quite inappropriate) sense of doom and decay. It is, of course, quite natural for any person to be thrown off balance by news of infection and disease, especially when the infection is portrayed almost relentlessly in the press as a death sentence. Fortunately, the facts are more reassuring. There is no question that

*Equivalent phrases include 'seropositive', 'body positive', 'AB positive', 'infected', 'having antibodies to HIV' and 'a positive antibody result'.

having AIDS is a very serious matter indeed. The early statistics concerning mortality from AIDS have been frightening. However, with the development of new treatment regimens in more recent times, people with AIDS are living longer, and with a better quality of life than was thought possible even two years ago. People with AIDS are not always the wasted, scarred and pitiful wretches that the papers would have us believe. The longest-diagnosed case I am aware of in England has had AIDS for almost seven years, and continues to thrive as an active businessman and traveller. Many of the courageous people whose ideas have contributed to this book have had AIDS for two or three years, and they maintain active and enjoyable lifestyles despite their diagnoses. Even those who are physically ill and sometimes incapacitated by their condition have often managed to maintain an enriching life with humour and honesty. That's why this book is called *Living with AIDS and HIV*. It might just as well have been called *Living* despite *AIDS and HIV*.

Facing the Crisis

This is not to deny that a diagnosis or a positive antibody result will, particularly in the early stages after diagnosis, create enormous difficulties and pose great questions that are often unavoidable. However, every crisis can be faced, and many patients have told me that they reached a certain point when they recognised that the decision about their future boiled down to this: 'I fight to live, or I give up and wait.' While this statement certainly has some validity, I think that it can only be made with certain qualifications.

First, there will be for some people times when their illness is such that they are too weak or tired to fight back. It is important to be aware of the power of illness—the power to drain stamina, motivation and especially hope. The patient who is seriously ill and faced by people saying 'Don't give up; you can get well if you fight and keep thinking positively about the future' may actually feel worse as a result. The good intentions of others may cause *guilt* to pile up on top of sickness. One of my patients called it 'the tyranny of positive thinking'. He felt guilty because his illness was so overwhelming at the time he was diagnosed that he simply couldn't find the energy for 'positive' thinking.

Second, many people have received a diagnosis in the context of difficult social, domestic and/or occupational conditions. It may be all very easy for people to say 'It's important for you to get out and enjoy yourself' (with the best of intentions, again), but such urging provides little comfort to persons who have no money or friends to enjoy themselves with. There may be no one they can 'safely' confide in regarding their medical status; their environment may be intolerant of their sexuality *and* their illness, making a helpful and supportive response to their condition well nigh impossible. In every case, there is a crucial need to be aware of the person's whole life before management advice is proffered.

Third, we each have the right to determine the manner of our own reaction to life-threatening circumstances. If the patient chooses not to fight, this decision (which may be more behavioural than intellectual) deserves just as much respect as decisions to do otherwise. In the same vein, people have the right to change their minds about what they want to do. Moral superiority has no place in this context.

Having said all this, there is one disturbing and avoidable side to the reactions of people towards diagnosed illness and infection that my patients have repeatedly stressed. They report that it is quite uncommon for doctors or other hospital staff to *encourage* their patients to have a sense of hope or determination to fight their illness. They have bemoaned the 'doom and gloom' approach of established medical authorities towards individuals with AIDS, and feel that the medical staff's sense of pessimism (or lack of optimism) towards them is a serious handicap in achieving a workable and helpful sense of perspective on their circumstances. Some patients have said that where medical staff do not reinforce and encourage their personal determination to live with AIDS, they feel more alone, afraid and perhaps even foolish for looking for a good quality of life and hope.

The Importance of Encouragement

My observations of many hundreds of people with HIV infection and disease suggest very clearly that the perspective a patient has on his or her illness or infection can play a significant part in the development of his or her condition. The documented experiences of people with cancer, showing that those who fight to live often have a longer, and better quality of, life (some even overcoming their illness completely), are mirrored to some extent in many people with AIDS. People with AIDS and HIV want to live, but some have reported that the reactions of people around them, including in some cases their doctors, often *encourage* them to see such desires as futile! These responses are not only unfair; they also represent bad medical practice. The courage and determination shown by patients, their lovers and their families deserves respect from all those involved in their care. Everyone concerned with HIV disease must appreciate that a statistical trend in mortality does not necessarily reflect the circumstances of the individual patient. Similarly, a sense of hope and a reinforcement of the will to fight for life is, for most patients I have spoken to,

Table 3.2 Typical patient questions following HIV results

Will the STD clinic inform my GP of my results? (Not if you don't want them to.)

Does having HIV infection affect my life insurance or medical insurance acceptability? (Only for future policies—present policies are unaffected.)

If I were to develop AIDS: (1) Would I be able to carry on working? (Hopefully, yes—your diagnostic illness might lay you low for a while, though.) (2) If I were unable to carry on working, would I be helped financially by the State? (Yes, you would be eligible for some benefits.)

Can HIV be passed on by kissing? (No.)

Is AIDS a long and unpleasant illness? (Not necessarily.)

Is there a phone number I can call if I get depressed or anxious? (Yes—ask your doctor or counsellor.)

Is one type of sexual activity safer than another? (Definitely yes—see Chapter 4.)

Is there any established link between AIDS/HIV and any other infectious diseases such as herpes, hepatitis, gonorrhoea and syphilis? (The viruses causing them can all be transmitted by certain sexual activities.)

If I have herpes, for example, with regular repeat attacks, will I be more at risk for AIDS? (Possibly.)

If I worry so much about my infection/disease that it causes me to require time off work, can I get a doctor's certificate without: (1) Being required to tell my GP? (You should be able to—from your STD clinic.) (2) Revealing the nature of my concern to my employer? (Yes.)

Are there ways of meeting other people who share my experience or anxieties, and can offer support? (Yes—ask your counsellor.)

If I stop having casual partners, will I reduce my risk of developing AIDS, or becoming sicker? (If you keep to safer sex, you can have as many casual partners as you like, though safer sex is possibly easier to maintain if you have fewer and steadier partners.)

If I become terminally ill with AIDS, will I be allowed or left to die alone and in pain? (No—no good doctor would allow this.)

information of the same importance as the nature of their diagnosis and methods of infection control.

Table 3.2 contains some of the questions that many patients have asked their doctors at the time they received news of their infection or disease. Doctors or counsellors should be able to help answer such questions (answers are given in parentheses).

TELLING OTHERS OF YOUR NEWS

Many people have spoken of the almost irrepressible urge to tell their news to everyone in the first hours or days after they have been told. The pressure to do so can seem overwhelming, especially if there is no one close with whom the news can be safely shared. However, it is crucially important for all patients to be advised to *tell no one* who is unaware of an attendance for results or diagnosis, for the time being at least. Even those who may be aware of a person's worries about health may not be prepared for the news, or to tolerate the reality of a diagnosis in their midst.

The reason for such caution is as follows. People who are only recently aware that they have AIDS, an AIDS-related illness or HIV infection are usually acutely self-conscious about their condition. They may be very easily upset by the shock, insensitivity or intolerance shown by others who are told about their circumstances. Often, bitter experience has shown that no matter how outwardly sympathetic and supportive people might be towards others (especially those in minority groups), their reactions to even old friends or colleagues with HIV infection or disease can vary widely. For example, many patients have confided in their employers about being seropositive and having AIDS, only to be immediately suspended, dismissed or prematurely 'retired' from work, irrespective of the evident lack of risk to colleagues, and the wishes and capacities of the patient. Sadly, many patients have reported that old and trusted friends have reacted to news about diagnoses with hysterical avoidance of touching, kissing, shared eating or drinking, or joint recreational activities. Perhaps worse than this, many 'friends' have immediately blabbed the news to others; what started as a shared confidence becomes public knowledge. Of course, the person who suffers most is the patient. Frequently, people diagnosed with AIDS are perfectly fit to work, yet the overreaction of employers and colleagues has meant that they can no longer do so. No work means no pay—this, in turn, means no money to pay mortgages, run cars, enjoy leisure, etc. What began as 'hot gossip' can become the beginning of a downward financial, social, psychological and then medical spiral, with all the imaginable miseries. Even where people have remained in work, the self-consciousness that goes with being the unstated focus of attention can cause intolerable stress.

This kind of scenario is unfortunately too common, and can result in severe disturbance and distress for persons at a time when they most require sensitive and trustworthy handling by those around them (in both the hospital and the community). Where sensitivity and discretion have *not* been provided, some people have felt sufficiently distressed to attempt suicide (a number have been tragically successful). It must be said that all of us in the community, no matter what our relationship to those with HIV disease, owe them respect and consideration in our dealings with them and concerning them. We would surely demand the same if it were us who were on the receiving end.

Deciding Who Should be Told

How, then, does one decide who should be told? The first issue is perhaps this: Who *needs* to know? It seems clear that persons providing health care which involves some degree of infection risk to themselves should have the opportunity to protect themselves effectively from this. Dentists, surgeons and GPs fall into this category, although it is hoped that they will all have taken care to ensure no possibility of infection to themselves (or their patients) by observing anti-hepatitis B precautions as a matter of *routine*. Worries may arise about such professionals choosing not to treat patients in view of their infection or, worse, about their informing other family members, employers or associates about the patient's condition. Where such doubts arise, the supervising hospital or clinic doctor or counsellor should be told of the patient's concern, so that they can organise health care by health staff who are appropriately informed about the infection and its control and who are reliably discreet and sympathetic. It is always important for people to be reassured that information concerning their health is only used by appropriate health professionals, and even then only when absolutely necessary. If you have any doubts about how the information is being handled (e.g. whether it is being passed to your GP without your consent), you should simply ask your attending hospital or clinic doctor about this.

Generally speaking, government guidelines about telling other health staff are aimed ultimately at preventing the spread of the infection. In most circumstances this means that only those hospital and/or clinic staff directly involved in patients' care are made aware of HIV infection or disease. The Government has made a point of informing all doctors in the United Kingdom that if they, or any other staff, allow information to be passed outside the sphere of personnel directly involved in patient care, they will be subject to the most severe disciplinary measures. Most health staff will be aware of the need to maintain confidentiality, although it is probably wise for patients to ask their physician *directly* what the options are, and to say clearly who they want told and not told. For example, some patients may not want their family doctor to be told, because they fear that the doctor may then tell other members of their family. In such cases these concerns should be made absolutely clear, preferably to more than one staff member. Staff may then be able to find another GP who is happy to take on the role of community doctor, thus avoiding fears of a leak in confidentiality to other family members.

As the infection may be transmitted from a pregnant mother to her unborn child, and this process may also lead to the development of severe disease in the infected mother, in relevant circumstances staff may wish to counsel spouses and, in particular, (potentially) pregnant partners of infected men about the risks they are facing. This may require divulging confidential information which may have a serious effect on the individual's relationship. For example, the infected partner may have to admit to being a drug user or a bisexual, or to having been sexually unfaithful. Solutions to such problems are never easy or straightforward. Again, it will require much serious and careful discussion with the counsellor and/or doctor so that all potential options are well aired in advance of others being told. It is important that all parties involved in the decision to tell or not spend sufficient time talking with the patient, so that avoidable mistakes are not made and unnecessary or prolonged distress is minimised. My own experience with such problems suggests that they are often 'no-win' situations. It is also necessary to avoid stereotyping these problems or applying rigid principles in response to them—every person is different and each has his or her own imperatives and issues to consider. A further point that *can* be made as a generalisation about such problems, however, is that it is usually better to deal with them sooner than later, especially where pregnancy is involved.

Talking about Sex

The issue of telling only those who need to know applies also to sexual activity. Sexual partners who are unaware that the patient is in a risk group for infection may need to be made aware of the 'safe sex' guidelines (discussed in Chapter 4). But how can a person with the infection bring such an issue up without scaring the (potential) partner off altogether? The answer is that it just takes practice and a little confidence.

The first rule in this situation is to be clear about what sexual activity you are prepared to enjoy. If you have decided that you wish to keep to the safest possible sex activities (e.g. mutual masturbation, 'dry' kissing, massage), it may be helpful to say something like 'I'm worried about the infections that are going round these days. Can we agree that coming *on* is good but coming *in* is bad?' An alternative: 'I'd really like to go to bed with you, but only if we stick to safe sex.' Such statements are not going to reveal that *you* are carrying the infection; they merely demonstrate your concern to avoid the spread of infection. And by bringing the subject up, you may be tremendously reassuring the other person, who is just as concerned about the risk of other sexual activities. More detailed discussion of safer sex will be found in Chapter 4.

Work

Regarding workmates or employers, HIV seropositives present absolutely *no risk* to them by being in the same environment, sharing coffee mugs, toilets and washrooms, etc. (see Chapter 4). However, even when such information is understood by colleagues, they may still feel that your presence among them is undesirable. Some patients have been suspended, fired, or involuntarily 'retired' or made 'redundant' as a result of pressure from colleagues' spouses, who irrationally fear for the welfare of their children. Some people have had to leave work because the presence of a person with HIV (with or without disease) is regarded as being bad for the image of the firm—it may scare clients or customers away, so the reasoning goes. Some people have had to leave work because their infection or disease has identified them as being homosexual or bisexual. In the case of teachers, for example, some have had to leave work in such circumstances because of the prevailing misconception that, irrespective of disease or infection, all homosexuals are child molesters. This is, of course, rubbish, but the power of this idea seems at present unassailable.

In view of such difficulties, it seems sensible to use the principle that if the employer and colleagues do not need to know, don't tell them. Absences from work for hospital or other check-ups may be explained in terms of treatment for some other, less emotive and prejudicial illness or reason. Where illness prevents the person from working for long periods, or if permanent retirement seems advisable, ask the doctor or counsellor about their experience in managing such situations. It may well be possible for a sickness pension to be facilitated without the reputation or confidentiality of the patient being tarnished. One of my patients with AIDS retired telling his firm that he had leukaemia—he was given a splendid leaving party and a handsome 'golden handshake'. Another retired saying that he had AIDS—no one would come to wish him farewell and good luck, and he received a miserable pension only after a great deal of argument (the stress of which he could ill afford).

It must also be said that many firms have shown the greatest possible compassion and sensitivity towards those of their staff who have become seropositive or developed disease from their infection. Fears of rejection have been countered by moving displays of acceptance and support from bosses and colleagues in such cases, including extended financial support and generous time off for medical reasons. The problem is that such understanding and beneficial responses are not often predictable.

Again, before any moves are made with regard to informing workmates, ask your doctor or counsellor whether they have any previous experience in dealing with the firm concerned. They may well have already established co-operative links with the company medical staff, who can provide discrete and confidential support for as long as it is required. Doctors should also be able to advise about particular medical issues that may be relevant to the work you do, such as the safety of particular vaccinations if your job involves travel.

Furthermore, before employers are informed, if this is at all necessary (and they should only be told if it is necessary, and with the patient's consent), it will be important to make sure that all the options are first considered, that all the medical replies to expected questions are rehearsed, and that 'fall-back' positions are clarified in the event of an adverse outcome. It may be helpful for a social worker to be alerted to the possible need for community back-up, financial benefits, etc., should things not work out with the employer.

Preparation

No matter who is told of the news, the preparation of clear and simple replies to expected questions is vital. Remember that in the popular imagination, as a result of much wilful distortion in sections of the popular media, AIDS and HIV infection or disease are widely regarded as somehow contagious, and it is this aspect of the patient's situation that will provoke the most alarm in most instances. Therefore, have a list of questions and answers prepared with the help of the doctor or counsellor, and *rehearse* them until you can give replies confidently. Such questions may well include those listed in Table 3.2. Topics raised by anxious friends, workmates and families include:

Are you infectious?
How is the infection spread?

Are you fit to work?
How much time will you need off work?
What special precautions or arrangements need to be made?
Who else knows about the situation?
Are you safe with children (will they catch anything off you)?
Is it safe for you to share the lavatory?
What can we do to help?

Many patients will want to turn to their family for support, understandably, although such a move may also be fraught with difficulties. For instance, the family members may be unaware that the patient is homosexual, or a drug user. Or they may be aware but disapproving. Important family members may avoid discussing the possibility of worsening health or death when the patient wants to. A very few patients have reported that telling their family has resulted in abuse and rejection, while others have said that although they desperately wanted to share the news, they were afraid for the effect on the health of elderly or ill parents.

Again, if the decision is made to inform family members, it is important to choose those who are most likely to be sympathetic, and to rehearse what will be said and how to say it. Perhaps those who are told will be able to offer useful advice on how to tell others whose reaction to the news will be less predictable. Issues relating to the involvement of families are discussed more fully in Chapter 6.

MANAGING THE FIRST FEW DAYS

The first thing to bear in mind is that *you are not alone*. There are many other people in your situation, and their experience can be put to your advantage. HIV infection and AIDS-related illnesses are no longer a novelty. Many doctors, health staff and community workers now have a wealth of experience in managing this problem, and their experience is an enormous asset. If you are dissatisfied with the quality of care you receive, first speak to them about it—there may be a simple misunderstanding of your needs and ways of communicating them.

Because so many people are in the same boat, many community agencies now exist to provide support and advice to those recently found seropositive or diagnosed. Your doctor or counsellor will be able to advise on which organisation may be of help to you, and it is probably a good idea at least to keep a note of how to contact them if you decide that you wish to know more in the future. Your counsellor or doctor should also help to provide a sense of perspective on the situation. I have often said to patients that it is most important to 'have

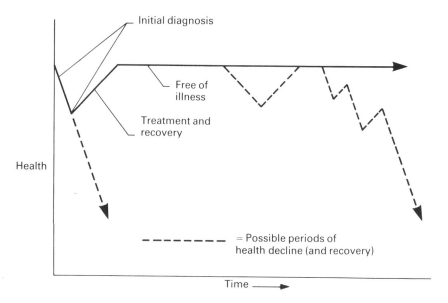

Figure 3.1   Natural history of AIDS (adapted with the permission of Dr A. Pinching)

a sense of history' about their situation. Having news of seropositivity does not mean that your whole life will never be the same again. For many people, all that's changed for them is that they have an extra piece of information about themselves. Physically, little else is different. Any changes in their lives will only involve particular sexual or other activities designed to maintain a good state of health.

For other people who are physically ill, a sense of history means recognising that many HIV-related diseases can now be treated effectively, and the physical quality of life will involve a period of recovery followed by extended periods of stability and freedom from illness. If the natural history of AIDS were to be shown as a graph, it would look like Figure 3.1. As the graph shows, most people can be successfully treated once they are diagnosed. They will then have a period free of illness—this period may be weeks, months or years. . . . As medical knowledge becomes more sophisticated, AIDS will, it is hoped, become completely manageable and non-fatal for all.

Confidence in one's doctors and health staff is very important, because it is important to have the confidence and encouragement to keep up hope and to 'hang on'. That is one reason why it is so important to have hospital and/or community staff who are prepared and able to talk to you about what is happening. Persons who are left alone to contemplate their circumstances, without sufficient information about their disease to be able to place it in a useful perspective, will almost always become depressed and resigned to death, irrespective of the medical facts of their own condition. So, never be afraid to ask about your condition—the news may be good!

Prognoses

If, at the time of diagnosis, you have been told that you can expect to live only for a finite period, remember that (a) the doctor may well be wrong, (b) medical help (e.g. a new drug) may be found in the meantime, and (c) you are not dead yet—there are still things you can do to make your life enjoyable and satisfying. In an earlier book I related the story of a clergyman who was told that he had only six months left to live. Immediately, he started a new appeal to reroof his church. 'Why are you doing this?' his amazed parishioners asked. 'You should be resting, taking it easy; you're very ill.' The clergyman replied that he *wanted* to do it, and not to do so would be like putting on his coat, getting a taxi and going to a party; then, when he arrived, not taking off his coat, talking to his friends, dancing, drinking, eating the delicious food and enjoying himself because the taxi would be coming to pick him up in a few hours and he would simply have to put his coat on again and go home!

Despite the clergyman's otherwise excellent example, I would suggest one further point in relation to handling such news:

> Don't overreact by trying to do everything at once. If you have been diagnosed with an illness that has laid you low, getting over that and managing the immediate practicalities associated with it (e.g. time off work, telling close and trusted others of the news) should be the first priority. Other decisions come later, when you're stronger. The rest of the book is concerned with these.

The same recommendation to take it easy and to delay making important or big decisions applies to those who are not seriously ill or who are seropositive without any symptoms. It is important to find a source of support and information, to meet them regularly (the counsellor should see you within a couple of days of your being told), to tell no one except your lover or whomever is closest and most reliable, and to gather information. Let yourself get used to the news (of course, this may take longer than just a few days). Big decisions come *after* you have understood fully what your infection means and what lifestyle changes are recommended—not before.

4

Practical Adjustments

WORK

Due to press reports [of my illness], everybody I work with knew about it and in my opinion it was the best thing that happened. My return to work was celebrated with champagne and cards. I had many visits in hospital from colleagues.

It is best not to tell your employer, because [if you do] you'll lose your job. If you are strong enough to work and not ill... don't tell your employer.

Don't tell anyone [at work] until there has been ample time to consider the possibilities and reactions.

... after talking to people at work I got a lot of Terrence Higgins Trust pamphlets from my STD clinic and gave them the pamphlets to read. But I only discussed it with those who mentioned my illness to me. I never brought the subject up first [in the past]. Now I do because the hysteria around the time of my diagnosis is not quite so bad.

I told my boss I was seropositive, because they knew I was gay, and had always shown me full support. I had been offered a partnership just two weeks before. My boss said he'd tell no one, but when his wife found out, she got all the other [directors'] wives together... as a result, the next day I was given two hours to leave the office. I have never been back. I have no career... and can't get another job, because I work in a small world and word will get around about why I had to leave when I was doing so well....

Experience has shown that it is desirable for people with HIV infection and/or disease to remain working wherever possible. There is certainly a financial advantage in doing so—not working for most of us means having a greatly reduced income at a time when financial flexibility can be very important. This, in turn, can lead to problems with keeping one's standard of living, accommodation and recreation. However, there is an equally important reason for staying in work if this is a realistic option: work provides a routine and a distraction away from the traumas of diagnosis or infection. After the initial period of coming to terms with the circumstances of infection, for most people there will come a time for getting on with their life—for starting to *live* with AIDS and/or HIV. Work is an important part of this.

The quotes above reflect the experiences of people who have told their work colleagues, and of some who have chosen to wait. In *all* cases, don't rush into telling anyone of news about HIV. To do so may result in very undesirable career consequences. If you have become aware of your infection status through your company doctor, it may be difficult to ensure that your circumstances remain confidential. Ask your doctor for advice. If the doctor is not able or equipped to offer constructive responses, get in touch with one of the community support organisations for HIV seropositives, or your Citizens' Advice Bureau; they have access to legal and financial advice that may be of help.

The abiding problem in informing anyone about personal HIV infection and/or disease is that reactions are unpredictable. Remember that HIV disease is not a 'glamorous' situation—it does not generate the same social sympathies as other serious or life-threatening illnesses that have from time to time preoccupied television viewers or newspaper readers. It is, instead, widely regarded still as a largely 'self-inflicted' plague that has 'innocent victims' alongside the major risk group of gay men. It is probably fair to say that, at the time of writing, social understanding is still in its formative stages—many people are unsure about how they should respond. AIDS is still a 'gay' and drug users' disease in their minds. As such, it has the additional stigma of minority sex and/or drug use attached to it, as do the patients. In consequence, all those afflicted must tread carefully lest they excite prejudice instead of support and understanding.

Again, deciding who to tell may be settled on a 'need to know' basis. In all cases, emphasise that the virus is completely non-infectious in routine person-to person social and occupational contact, and that no 'special' precautions or facilities (e.g. separate lavatories) are required. Before telling anyone, however, rehearse your statements so that you are as comfortable as possible in discussing the facts of your infection. If you look and sound confident, your employers and colleagues will be more confident too.

In the context of work, there may be many good reasons for telling others of the situation. For some people, work colleagues are their closest associates; friendship may be the reason. Others may have a personal interest in their work—they may own their own business, or be the person in charge. Others may have a job that requires travelling—they may need 'live' vaccinations if they travel in certain parts of the world where particular diseases are still seen. Or they may be travelling to work in a country where a certificate providing evidence of no HIV infection is required before entry (e.g. Saudi Arabia and the United Arab Emirates). They may be applying for a job where an anti-HIV screening test is a mandatory part of their medical examination, or this test may have recently been introduced in annual medical examinations. Whatever the reason, if the subject is to be discussed, some issues will have to be clarified *in advance*.

First, *who* precisely will be told. The experience of one of the patients quoted above indicates that even if only one or two are informed, they may well tell others at home or elsewhere (imagine the gossip value in the pub!).

Second, the responses of employers may well reflect an additional concern (e.g. about the cost to their company in time or money lost through illness, or a reduced ability of the patient to effectively make important decisions). To answer such concerns effectively, it will be necessary to have as many facts available as possible, so that decisions made regarding your future are based soundly upon known circumstances—not misleading speculation.

A third issue concerns the effect such news may have on your colleagues if they know your circumstances. We have seen (above) how one person with AIDS received a degree of acceptance and support from workmates that he didn't dare hope for; but for many the situation has been very much different. Again, take care in telling. If you have good reasons for thinking that life will be made unmanageable at work through the reactions of workmates, it may be better to leave and attempt to find other work after all. Patients frequently report that where they have been seriously physically ill for some time, the stress of work is actually counterproductive. But leaving for a quieter life must be balanced against the usefulness of a regular income and a routine distraction from illness or infection.

In order to make the decision about whether to stay at work or not easier to reach, try making up a 'pros and cons' table. On one side ('pros') list all the advantages of staying employed or working. These might include having a regular income, having a routine, having a distraction from your health situation and keeping in touch with friends or the outside world. Then, on the 'cons' side, list the disadvantages you can think of (which will depend to a large extent on the severity of your illness). These might include difficulties with the reactions of colleagues, problems with organising time off work, the unwanted extra stress arising from work, etc. If you know of others at your workplace who have been identified seropositive or received a diagnosis of HIV disease, perhaps you could ask them about their experience in managing this issue. They may know of particular redundancy or sickness benefits that your firm is prepared to offer. A typical pros and cons table is shown in Table 4.1.

Table 4.1 Pros and cons of staying at work

Pros	Cons
Regular income	Stress with demands of work
Routine activity	Uncertainty over future ability to work
Satisfaction	Difficulties with the reactions of colleagues
Seeing friends regularly	Physical limitations

After learning about your HIV infection, it may be helpful to take a short break from work, if this is possible. This time can then be used to come to terms with the news, and to clarify what to do next. Discussion with selected close friends, the clinic or hospital doctor or counsellor may be particularly helpful at this time. It is important to avoid rushing any decisions of this nature—time spent carefully now may save much distress later.

SAFER SEX

> My libido was shattered for a time after my diagnosis. However, I realised that it was important to recognise that my sexuality had not come to an end.

> Since being diagnosed, I find I have become extremely screwed up, *not* about my sexuality, but about sex. Sex had never bothered me before—homosexuality has always been normal for me. It is very difficult to discuss safe sex with prospective partners. When certain activities are taken out of sex, such as sucking and fucking, little is left.

> I've had safe sex with a person who knew of my illness and it was disastrous. I've since had very safe sex with someone

who doesn't know and it was very satisfactory, but I'm starting to worry about whether he has a right to know.

I see safe sex as something that is *not* an option. I do not want anyone else to go through what I've gone through.

Safe sex is great. I don't have to worry about catching anything, and so I'm more relaxed and can actually enjoy sex more.

You get used to it.

The AIDS scare has made us closer. We talk about things more. We don't cruise any more. We take more care in our sex life. I miss some of the things I used to do, but I wouldn't want to pass HIV on.

My wife and I want kids, but we know we can't have them now. I do sometimes worry that on top of everything else [arising from my haemophilia] this may be the last straw and she may want to leave.

Safer sex, together with prevention of needle-sharing, is at present the *only* way in which the HIV epidemic will be stopped. For many people, this preventative measure is the biggest challenge they will face in the context of their infection. However, sex is for many seropositive people more than just a matter of pleasure and/or orgasms. Sex also implies affirming one's sexuality, having children, meeting people and making friends, and just being a part of contemporary society. A recommendation to limit one's sexual expression, therefore, is also seen by many as a recommendation to deny these other vital ingredients of a full and happy life.

Of course, no one has the power to forcibly prevent people from doing whatever they want, sexually. The decision to follow safer sex guidelines is theirs and theirs alone. Some people will not take this decision. That is why the number of seropositive persons continues to increase, and why the number of people with AIDS grows every day. Perhaps part of the reason for this is that the guidelines are seen as moralistic, or 'antigay', or antifun. Perhaps another part of the reason is that many seropositives are simply unaware that they have the infection, and therefore see no need to adjust their sexual repertoire. And, of course, some people will not bring the subject of safer sex up with prospective sexual partners, because they fear being rejected sexually, emotionally or socially. Yet it is significant that the first safer sex guidelines were published by members of the largest risk group for HIV—homosexual men. And for many, many people who have adopted the safer sex guidelines, they have come to represent not a denial of their sexuality but an *affirmation* of it. It is important to remember throughout that safer sex does not mean that you have to have less sex—just *safer* sex.

The safer sex guidelines currently recommended are as follows.

1. *Avoid* (unprotected) anal and vaginal intercourse. *It is safest to avoid intercourse altogether.* However, if this is simply unacceptable, it is important always to use a strong condom *together with a water-based lubricant* such as KY Jelly or a spermicide. But using condoms and lubricants does *not* make intercourse 100 per cent safe—there is always a risk that the condom may tear.

   The logic of this precaution is as follows: anal intercourse frequently causes tearing of the delicate lining of the rectum (the mucosa), resulting in bleeding. Furthermore, the delicate mucosal lining of both the rectum and the cervix are known to contain T cells (probably from local secretions and/or the uterus in women). These cells may become infected with HIV during sexual contact (e.g. from infected semen). Therefore, using a barrier such as a condom may prevent the passage of HIV from infected semen and/or from infected anal or genital secretions (it is thought that the inserter may acquire HIV from the passive partner if he has small areas of infection in his urethra). Additionally, condoms are known to help reduce the incidence of other sexually transmitted diseases (STDs), such as herpes, gonorrhoea and syphilis. It is widely considered possible that catching such diseases either just before or during HIV infection may lead to active HIV disease, so using a condom gives extra protection if anal or vaginal intercourse cannot be avoided.

   If condoms are being used, here are some further important points to remember.

   ● They may take some getting used to, so practise putting them on before you need to.

   ● Don't use oil-based lubricants with the condom (e.g. Vaseline)—they dissolve the condom very quickly. Water-based lubricants are the only safe ones. Some spermicides contain an agent called 'Nonoxinol 9' which is known to destroy HIV on contact (e.g. if the condom tears).

   ● Don't use saliva or spit as your lubricant—it doesn't remain slippery for long enough.

   ● Don't reuse the condom—use a new one each time you have intercourse.

● During intercourse, check to make sure that the condom is still on properly (they can slip off sometimes!).

● Once you have 'come', or ejaculated, pull out of your partner straight away while holding on to the condom at the base of your penis, as the semen could seep out into the partner when the penis has gone limp.

2. *Avoid oral-genital and oral-anal sex* (fellatio, or 'sucking'; cunnilingus, or 'rimming'). While it seems unlikely that HIV could be passed on by such activities, except possibly if there is bleeding, or cuts and sores in the mouth, it is clear that other STDs can be passed on in these ways. It is important to remember that HIV has been found in body fluids such as semen, pre-ejaculatory fluid (the clear lubricating fluid from the erect penis) and urine, so such activities must always be considered risky.

3. *Do not share vibrators, dildos or 'toys'.* They are perfectly safe when used only by one person, but, if shared, infected body fluids may be passed on.

4. *Sex involving large amounts of body fluids, such as 'water sports', can be very risky,* particularly if urine gets into eyes, cuts or the mouth. Although HIV is considered uninfectious in urine, other infectious agents such as cytomegalovirus may be spread in this way and thus create additional health problems. If these areas can safely be avoided, sex should be safe.

5. *Avoid sex in groups.* If more than one partner is involved, there may be pressure to take unwanted risks, so it is easiest and safest to have safer sex only with one other person (at a time!).

6. *Avoid high alcohol- or drug-taking before and during sex.* They may make sex more relaxing and enjoyable, but both alcohol and drugs affect judgement (including the ability to say 'no' politely and firmly!). It is particularly important to avoid injecting drugs with a syringe that has been used by others.

7. *Stay away from those places where there may be 'pressure' to have sex.* It can be difficult to keep your resolve about safe sex if you are around people who don't think the same way, or who are being obvious about their own lack of concern for good health. If recreation has been associated with particular (meeting) places where sex is available, it may be helpful to try elsewhere, where the pressures aren't the same. Alternatively, join groups that publicly endorse and encourage safer sex, so that opportunities for sexual activity arise in the context of mutual understanding about what is and is not acceptable. Sex can then be relaxing, because you both know what is safe and are both prepared to stick to what is safe.

8. *Discuss safer sex with all prospective partners*. A common fear of talking about safer sex with someone is that he or she will be scared off or will make fun of you for bringing the subject up. This fear is especially felt by people having casual encounters or having a sexual experience for the first time with someone new. In particular, people may feel that, by bringing the subject of safe sex up, they will identify themselves as being seropositive, making otherwise quite promising opportunities for (sexual) relationships highly unlikely. Of course, what is said to the prospective partner about one's infection is up to the individual, but there is no obvious reason why having HIV should enter into the discussion. (Many people who have developed a close and trusting relationship involving safer sex have said at a later stage that they felt deceitful in not making the fact of their infection clear to their lover. This will be discussed in Chapter 6.)

The fact is that using a condom and lubricant is advisable protection against giving and receiving STDs, and avoiding pregnancy. Heterosexual men and women could even say that they needed to use one because they had a bad case of thrush! Where it is clear to both partners that one or both belong to a high-risk group for HIV infection, discussion can be more straightforward. One can be honest about wanting to avoid the spread of HIV. Such an approach may be very reassuring to the partner who didn't know how to bring the subject up—perhaps because he or she was afraid of a rejection! Partners in these groups who are prepared to dismiss such precautions may be seen as poor candidates for sex, and for deeper involvement.

The important thing is to be clear in your own mind about what for you is and is not acceptable sexual behaviour, and to make this clear to the other person. An absence of ambiguity will set the scene for a more relaxed sexual experience, especially if you have rehearsed your explanations beforehand.

So, what really is safer sex? Safer sex techniques that avoid any risk of exposure to HIV (and other STDs) include any sexual activities that involve *no* body fluids such as blood, semen or urine coming in contact with broken skin or mucosal surfaces. The following activities are safe in these circumstances:

● (Mutual) masturbation to orgasm/ejaculation.

● Kissing—if there are no cuts, sores or infections in your mouth and on your tongue.

● Massage and 'body-rubbing' (sweating presents no infection problem).

● Using vibrators, dildos and 'toys'—but they must not be shared.

● Any other variations and activities that do not break the skin or allow the passage of fluids on or into vulnerable areas (mucosal and broken skin surfaces).

The question is: *How can sex be exciting with so many restrictions?* The answer is that it can be exciting but it may take practice and determination—changing such an important habit this much is never easy. There is, however, a side to safer sex that has not yet been considered—*the mind*! If you think about it, so much of sex is in the mind. Physical acts usually only approximate the fantasies we may have about sex with others. But fantasies work both ways—they can excite us *and* our partners, if we learn how to communicate them effectively.

Clearly, it may be difficult for many people to discuss their sexual fantasies and desires with someone they don't know or, more importantly, trust—for example, on the first 'date'. It can be difficult to make one's self so vulnerable to another if the encounter is casual or in uncertain circumstances. Perhaps it is for this reason that many people who have in the past been used to mainly casual sex have changed to more regular or longer-term relationships. For them, at least, sex has become part of a trusting relationship. One couple put it this way:

> We had always cruised before he was diagnosed—I suppose we were after something special or exciting. It was superficial and, to some extent, exciting, but we soon saw that it was dangerous. We made a decision ... to look after each other. We found that by looking to our relationship [of five years] again, we found what had attracted us [to each other] again. We talked in a different way ... I suppose we fell in love again. It is different, and we both miss parts of what we used to do, but not that much. If we do, we talk about it and that usually results in a good evening! The change in our lives has been worth it, for us, anyway.

It should be emphasised that sex means different things to different people, and the experience of one or even most people or couples should not be held up as the standard by which all other sexual expressions should be judged. For many seropositives, casual encounters remain their preferred sexual outlet, and they have been able to maintain this lifestyle and incorporate safe sex within it. The statement of Max, an American, is instructive:

> ... I've developed a real revived interest in dating and flirtations. Unlike some, I don't feel deprived by safer sex—in fact, the opposite. I celebrate safe sex as an opportunity for me to continue to express myself as a sexual being. At the same time, I can explore the wonders of intimacy and the many non-sexual elements of my identity.... Besides, it's fun. More than ever, I like to feel attractive and warm and sexy and desirable. It's important for us people with AIDS, and people without AIDS as well, to remember that sex and touching are still in our repertoire.

The point of this section is merely to indicate that where people have become comfortable in communicating their special delights to others, safer sex has become (usually to their surprise) as much, or even more, of a pleasure as before, because they no longer fear its consequences. Where trust and confidence in one's partner is a feature of sexual activity, the depth of sexual feeling can be greater and, many of my patients have stated, more satisfying.

For those who do not have relationships, or who have chosen not to be active sexually with others, a healthy sex life can still be maintained. Masturbation does not, contrary to the opinion of our Victorian forebears, lead to physical decline or loss of vital faculties, or even of 'moral fibre'! Masturbation is healthy and enjoyable, and can provide a welcome relief from a variety of stresses and needs. Above all, it is *normal*. It is certainly a good way of using one's imagination, and using books, pictures and other facilities can make it even more enjoyable. As one of my patients with AIDS cheerfully reported a few weeks after he had been diagnosed:

> I made the choice to become celibate after a lifetime of rather rampant sex. I hired one of those video machines, got a supply of rather pornographic tapes, and have been pleasuring myself very enjoyably ever since.

This person eventually felt a need to touch other people sexually again, and has since had a series of safer sex encounters.

An interesting footnote to this section is supplied by Peter, a person who has recently been diagnosed with AIDS after having known of his HIV infection for many months. A charming, warm and thoughtful man, he made the point that spending less time on organising a casual sex life meant more time for other things.

> Life has genuinely become more interesting. It's funny really, but sex has somehow been put in perspective. It takes time, but I like the change and all the new things in my life that there was no time for before.

INFECTION CONTROL

This section is designed to inform seropositive people and their carers about how to avoid passing their infection on to others. We have already discussed safer sex; the discussion now turns to other areas of life in which there is a *remote* possibility of virus transmission.

The first point to consider is that HIV is a particularly vulnerable virus. Its thin, buttery envelope gives it very little protection against the 'outside' world. This means not only that it is easily destroyed when outside the incubating protection of the body—it is also a very difficult virus to acquire. In fact, studies of the spread of the virus from around the world are unanimous in identifying the following definite routes of transmission:

1. Invasive sexual contact.
2. Injecting drug use.
3. Donated and injected blood, blood products and other body fluids (e.g. sperm).
4. Intrauterine passage from mothers to neonates, and to babies through infected breast milk.
5. Exposure of open skin wounds to large amounts of infected blood and body fluids.

Exposure of infected blood and body fluids to mucosal surfaces apart from the vagina and rectum (e.g. eyes and mouth) may carry some risk but this is not proven.

For many years now, researchers have been very concerned to see whether there were any indications of HIV transmission by other routes. Families of adults and children with HIV and AIDS have been scrupulously assessed for long periods of time. The good news is that, apart from the risk routes described, *there is absolutely no risk of infection by any other route*. Contact within families, especially among young children and their parents, has been shown to be safe. So conventional social and work contact creates no risk.

Despite this reliable finding, public reaction to HIV indicates that such information has yet to be widely appreciated. For instance, the revelation that the virus has been found in saliva generated great concern about the potential dangers associated with kissing, spitting, biting, etc. Children with haemophilia and HIV infection were shunned at school (or asked to stay at home), and parents of other pupils kept their children at home for fear that they would catch the virus in the classroom or in the playground. Many patients have reported that family members have kept them away from nieces, nephews, grandchildren, young brothers and sisters, because of such anxieties. One patient with AIDS was welcomed back to work after his diagnosis, only to find that he had a special lavatory all to himself. (Actually, he was quite pleased about not having to queue to use it any more!) There have been numerous reports of gay men being banned from pubs and clubs; one professional colleague even found herself under strident interrogation from a landlord who became terrified of the risk she supposedly represented—he discovered that she was renting his room while attending a conference on AIDS!

We are all probably aware of the types of press headlines that highlight and distort the risks of infection:

AIDS MAN BITES TWO COPS

AIDS HORROR ON QE2

COURTROOM CLEARED FOR KILLER-PLAGUE CARRIER

The problem with such wilful distortions of the risks of infection is that they contribute to and maintain public ignorance of the facts. It is no surprise, therefore, that fears of infection from everyday social, domestic and work contact are so prominent (and often so unnecessarily destructive). A typical example concerned the elderly parents of a person with PGL. They were desperately concerned for their son, and felt that the most constructive practical help they could provide was to have him at their home in the country each weekend; there they could look after him away from the city pressures he constantly faced. However, as no one had given them clear guidance on the risk of infection from their son, they would burn his bedsheets each Sunday evening after he had returned to his own home. This was expensive (they are pensioners) and created much guilt in them both— they saw their actions as unfair and distancing, yet they felt that they had no choice. Imagine their relief when they were told that their son's sheets could be washed normally in a hot household washing cycle— along with their other clothes!

Another young man who acquired his HIV when working in Africa took exceptional care over passing it on to others. A popular and attractive person, he had many friends and was regularly invited out to dinner. He would take two plastic bags with him. One contained a complete set of crockery and cutlery, which he would eat and drink with. He would then put the used utensils in his bag, take them home and scrub them in boiling water! The other bag contained two rags and a bottle of disinfectant. Whenever he visited his hosts' lavatory, he would use these to scrub and disinfect it to a standard that would be the envy of many hospital operating theatres. (Needless to say, he was often invited back on a weekly basis!)

Such overreaction is entirely misplaced. Sensible household hygiene measures are all that's necessary to prevent the spread of infection in *all* cases. HIV *cannot* be spread through sharing crockery, cutlery, lavatories and bathrooms, towels or bed linen, by shaking hands, by using doorknobs, by kissing, hugging or cuddling. It naturally makes good sense for all people to keep to the following guidelines:

Wash your hands regularly, and keep yourself clean by bathing daily, where this is possible.

Wash all utensils in dishwashing detergent and water hot enough to require wearing rubber gloves.

Use different cloths for cleaning the kitchen and the bathroom, and use different cloths for cleaning work surfaces and floors.

Wash hands after handling pets and litter trays (in fact, it is best to clean litter trays and animal spills while wearing rubber or plastic gloves). As pets may harbour organisms that could be harmful to a person with AIDS, they should not be allowed to lick your face, and care should be taken to minimise their contact with other animals. Finally, make sure that they are regularly inoculated and kept clean and healthy.

Make sure that meat (particularly poultry) is defrosted and cooked thoroughly—poorly prepared meats may harbour bacteria or other potentially dangerous organisms.

Clean your refrigerator regularly, disposing of stale or old food on a regular basis. Use soap and water to dispose of any moulds that you find growing there!

Wear gloves for gardening.

Wear rubber or plastic gloves for cleaning up blood, vomit, semen or excrement spillages, and wash 'contaminated' areas of skin with warm soapy water.

Body fluid spillages should ideally be cleaned up with paper towels, and the towels should then be flushed down the lavatory. Affected household surfaces can then be disinfected by washing them in a 10 per cent solution of household bleach in water. Dirty fabrics can be safely cleaned by a conventional hot wash cycle in a domestic washing machine or commercial laundrette and then dried in a conventional home dryer. Where clothes and fabrics are heavily contaminated with faeces, urine or other bodily fluids, it makes sense to wash these separately—where any contamination is light, other non-contaminated clothes may be safely included in this wash.

- Any cuts, grazes or other skin lesions (e.g. eczema) should be covered in a waterproof dressing until healed (especially if close physical contact is anticipated).

- Where blood or other infected bodily fluid is splashed into the eyes or mouth, or on to the skin, of other persons, the affected surfaces should be washed out or off immediately with copious amounts of water. Skin surfaces should be washed with soapy water and rinsed.

- Ordinary household rubbish should be disposed of normally in tied plastic bags.

- Used dressings, tampons, sanitary towels and tissues can be disposed of down the lavatory or in securely tied rubbish bags.

- Avoid sharing toothbrushes and razors (see below).

In addition to these guidelines, other sources of risk must be considered. These apply to all persons within risk groups for HIV infection whether they know themselves to be seropositive or not:

1. Do not donate blood, body fluids or organs. Any organ donor cards being carried should be destroyed, and blood donations should cease.

2. Think very carefully about becoming or (if you are) remaining pregnant. Pregnant seropositive women run a higher than normal risk of developing severe disease from their infection, owing to the effects of pregnancy on the immune system. It is also tragically certain that infants born from seropositive mothers run a grave risk of being infected with HIV, and about 50 per cent are likely to die of AIDS within 12 months.

3. Having ears pierced, acupuncture, tattoos and being shaved in a barber's shop: all of these procedures may be risky for a couple of reasons. First, there may be small amounts of blood spilled or left on the instruments used. With such procedures, the risk of HIV infection is virtually zero, although *other* infections (such as hepatitis B) may be spread in such ways. Second, sterilisation of instruments cannot be fully guaranteed, and if large numbers of customers are being seen, there may be a slight degree of risk. Better to be safe and avoid such procedures.

4. Sharing toothbrushes and 'wet' razors in the home is best avoided. Again, the degree of risk is very small, and there is *no evidence* for the spread of HIV from such activities. However, observing such precautions has the advantage of bringing peace of mind and confidence that no risk whatsoever from other infections is being posed to others.

Total health care and infection control involves considering other persons who may, through their work, be exposed to infected body fluids.

Elsewhere in the book, the issue of informing one's general practitioner has been raised, and it is appropriate to do so again here. It is fair to say that medical opinion is still somewhat divided over the patient's (and the diagnosing physician's) responsibility to inform the GP about the infection. Overall, it is a wise precaution to have some form of medical supervision—the degree of which depends on the severity of illness—from a community doctor. But the decision about which doctor provides such supervision must be the patient's. If there are objections to having the family doctor involved, perhaps because he or she knows other family members who are unaware of the situation, then the clinic or hospital (or perhaps a community agency concerned with HIV) should be able to give advice on alternative practitioners who are prepared to offer necessary monitoring and support.

Similarly, dentists may be vulnerable to infection through particular dental procedures, even though they should be observing infection-control guidelines that avoid such a possibility *in all cases*, whether identified seropositives or not. At the time of writing, no cases of dentists becoming infected with HIV as a result of their work have been recorded, although dentist colleagues inform me that some surgical procedures do result in unintended skin puncturing by wires, etc. The fact is that a finger-prick from a piece of fine wire would almost certainly involve too small an amount of any HIV-infected fluid to be infectious, but at the same time, other dental procedures may involve larger amounts of blood (extractions, for example) which may splash into the dentist's eyes or mouth. They should, therefore, be given the opportunity to prepare themselves sufficiently against such a possibility. For this reason, dentists should be informed of the HIV infection of their patient. Dentists who are prepared to work in such conditions will be known to most hospitals, clinics and community agencies.

A Word about HIV-infected Schoolchildren

School-age children with HIV are from two main groups: (1) haemophiliacs who have used batches of Factor VIII and Factor IX (blood-clotting agents extracted from donated blood) infected with the virus; and (2) children whose mothers have been infected with HIV, and who have passed the infection on during pregnancy or birth, or through their breast milk.

It must be stressed that, of all the identified cases of HIV infection world-wide, *there is no evidence of any cases resulting from casual personal contact in schools or close (non-sexual) contact in families.*

Some children will, of course, have more physical and behavioural difficulties than others with regard to controlling bodily secretions, and in such cases (e.g. the neurologically impaired and developmentally handicapped) infection-control procedures should be well understood and rehearsed by the relevant teachers and nurses (see below). For all cases, however, 'normal' childhood habits such as thumb-sucking, chewing of pens or pencils, and placing objects in the mouth present no health risk to other children.

Where children are identified as having behavioural difficulties, (e.g. biting or fighting), an assessment of their individual circumstances can be made to determine their vulnerability and the degree of risk they may pose to others. In some cases special precautions may be required to protect the children concerned from harm.

Children infected with HIV may be more vulnerable to catching common childhood infections, such as measles, cold sores (herpes simplex) and chickenpox. They may also suffer more complications from them because of their lowered ability to fight off infections. Where such risks may be present, the physician in charge of the child's medical care will make appropriate recommendations about his or her management. As, in some cases, mental functions may become impaired as a result of a child's infection, it is important for staff to be alert to any changes in intellectual performance.

With the range of subjects that children may take at school, *normal* safety and hygiene precautions should be followed at all times. Parents, staff and other children can rest assured that courses involving shared wind musical instruments, and mouth-to-mouth resuscitation in first aid, pose no extra hazard to other pupils or to those with HIV infection.

Finally, as with all persons with HIV infection or HIV disease, the right of personal confidentiality is paramount with HIV-infected schoolchildren. The 'need to know' principle applies with children as with adults, and should be discussed with the supervising physician before any other personnel are involved.

HEALTH BOOSTING

The emphasis of this book is designed to enable the reader to achieve a practical and mental mastery over the circumstances of infection and/or disease. However, much of the advice so far seems to concern what *not* to do. We shall, therefore, now examine some of the things that many people have found it helpful to do in order to help themselves.

Living with AIDS and HIV means adopting a positive strategy of action rather than a passive strategy of waiting for the worst. This section contains tips, from many people who have lived with their infection or disease, that seem to work. It is important to remember, however, that the suggestions made are not touted as *cures*—rather, they are offered as ways for developing a working tolerance for the disruptions that infection and disease can bring. First, consideration of sensible health measures will be made.

Just as conventional standards of hygiene in the home, work and recreational environments apply to all people (whether seropositive or not), so do suggestions for maintaining good health and fitness. For example, it makes sense for all people to observe the following recommendations.

Ensure that You Have Sufficient Sleep on a Regular Basis

Sleep helps the body to 'recharge its batteries'—if we don't get enough, we simply drain our resources. There are times when one can't get enough sleep, perhaps because of a period of intense socialising or entertainment, and there is always the issue of balancing pleasure to be gained from such activities against the disappointment of not being involved. It is, after all, important to enjoy one's life whenever possible, irrespective of circumstances. The sensible course is to do as much as one can without doing too much and getting overtired. If there are times when doing other things gets in the way of a regular sleep cycle, make sure that there is time made later to catch up on sleep lost. As one of my patients put it:

> My life is a continual balancing act. For most of the time I do all those things that are good for me. I sometimes do things that are probably bad for me. I can't be sensible *all* the time and enjoyment of life, without putting others at risk, is the most important factor for me. I am in control of my fate and whatever treatments, therapies and lifestyles I choose can help me stay that way.

Get Regular Exercise

Don't overdo it, however. One needs to acquire a tolerance for exercise (rather in the same way that one acquires a tolerance for alcohol), and many people will be too physically weak to do too much for a while after initial diagnosis. However, it is a good idea to at least plan a regimen for daily exercise. This regimen should include, if possible, a *range* of exercise activities, so that future workouts are not limited by the availability of local facilities or a progressive illness that may cause discomfort or embarrassment. David, a member of the People with AIDS Group, explains:

> I found it very hard to take up swimming. Now, my KS is so advanced that I am too embarrassed to do so in public. I wish I had been warned—it didn't occur to me at the time—I might have taken up something else which I could still be doing.

People who are confined temporarily to a bed or a chair could perhaps begin by spending a few minutes daily on isometric exercises, which are not very physically involving. As health and stamina gradually improve, the range of exercises performed can be expanded. The benefits are obvious—improved muscle tone and physical stamina will result with regular practice. However, there are other benefits too—many researchers have found that regular exercise helps to lift depression and a general sense of well-being results. A regular exercise programme helps create a routine in the day, and a distraction from persisting worries for a while at least. Perhaps as important as these is knowing that by exercising in your own time each day, you are developing a form of *mastery* over your circumstances. An important point to remember is: take it gradually but consistently.

Learn to Eat a Healthy Diet

The issues of moderation and regularity relating to exercise also apply to what you eat. Many people with AIDS and HIV have taken up new diets in the belief that they can boost their immune efficiency by eating certain foods and avoiding others. This may be the case, but it is important to bear in mind that no diet will *cure* AIDS. Diet regimens are an ideal platform for faddist fanatics and fashion freaks, and while there has been no shortage of suggestions for AIDS diets from protagonists world-wide, the problem with the many diets that are publicised and taken up with an often religious fervour lies in their being unproven scientifically. However, this does not necessarily mean that they are not helpful. Indeed, it seems unfair and narrow-minded to dismiss nutrition programmes that may hold considerable promise in maintaining good health and that may even have restorative properties for people with significant illness. It just means that there is no reliable evidence that they can do what their authors may claim. It is also important to remember that one particular diet may not suit everyone's needs. A diet that seems helpful for one person may be unhelpful or even dangerous for another. Therefore, any new diet that is taken on in response to HIV infection or disease should be fully discussed with your physician and a nutritionist first.

Many people with HIV and/or AIDS have taken on macrobiotic, vegan, vegetarian, 'anticancer' and other diets, and most report that their new food regimen makes a significant difference to the way they feel. Grahame, one of the stalwarts of our People with AIDS Group, has embraced a naturopathic regimen and managed to maintain it for two years. He says he feels very well, and he certainly appears to be in the peak of health and condition. His diet excludes any red meat, pepper, caffeine, alcohol, sugar, and artificial flavourings or preservatives. However, one of the other group stalwarts, David, enjoys his traditional diet of fried eggs, beans, chips, chocolate bars and other foods denounced by Grahame. They both report feeling well, and both look equally healthy.

Perhaps the answer to the question 'Which diet is best?' is that it matters less what you eat than what you *feel* about what you eat. Persons making large changes in their approach to food will be making a commitment to their health that will probably take in other changes as well. For one thing, many health-oriented diets take substantial amounts of time from the day for food preparation. Many diets are designed as a part of a whole-person approach to health, and will include an active commitment to exercise, meditation, etc. In view of this, the statement of one person with AIDS, that ' . . . no matter what you get involved in, the involvement itself will help', is very significant. Personal dietary management is yet another step forward in achieving mastery and personal control over one's health circumstances. Even if your diet doesn't change, the active personal decision not to change it is an important first step in developing a self-control perspective on your new health status.

Some good news has recently emerged from one scientific analysis of the effects of an organic vegetarian (macrobiotic) diet on lymphocyte counts in a population of men with AIDS. They were found to be stable or slowly increasing over time. If more data were available on the precise effects of particular diets, confidence in them would undoubtedly increase and the faith of a few 'pioneers' would perhaps be justified.

For those who are less inclined to adopt more stringent dietary responses to their health circumstances, it is important to remember that sensible eating is very necessary. This means that you eat fresh vegetables and fruit; that meats should be fresh, thoroughly defrosted and cooked; and that meals should be taken *regularly*. 'Fast food' should not be your staple diet, and diet should be balanced—i.e. should contain sufficient levels of carbohydrates, proteins, vitamins, minerals, fibre and the other essential things that make for healthy eating. A further important point is that you should eat what you enjoy: just because food is good for you does not mean that it is boring—it can be delicious. Take time to learn what is best, and then some time to learn how to prepare it. Your new habit will be doing you much good, and be a pleasure.

Some foods are best avoided by people with HIV infection and/or disease. For example, non-pasteurised milk and milk products have, in the past, been associated with *Salmonella* infection—this infection can lead to dangerous complications in a person with AIDS. Similarly, organically grown food, which has been fertilised with animal or human waste, may contain some degree of hazard unless cooked before eating. As a general guide, a diet plan has been prepared by the nutrition department at St. Mary's Hospital, and is reproduced in Table 4.2. Vegetarians may exclude meats from the plan. In addition to following the general outline of the plan, it may also be helpful to take a course of multivitamin supplements to ensure that essential vitamins are consumed regularly (there is no need to overdo this— check with your doctor for the best amount).

Finally, the Health Education Council has produced an excellent booklet entitled *Guide to Healthy Eating*, which contains a wealth of useful detailed information on diet and maintaining optimum body weight. Copies are available free of charge from The Health Education Council, 78 New Oxford Street, London WC1A AH.

Reduce Recreational Drug Use

From the earliest days of the HIV epidemic, the use of recreational drugs such as nitrites or 'poppers' was thought to be one of the possible causes of AIDS, mainly because using such chemicals creates temporarily lowered immune efficiency. We now know that these drugs, which are used to enhance the sensation of orgasm, are not the cause of AIDS, but the significance of their immune-depressant effect remains.

Other researchers have noticed an association between immune suppression and other drugs, such as tobacco and even alcohol. The essential point, therefore, is that any drugs should be taken only *in moderation*. Indeed, it is probably best to avoid their use altogether. However, lest any puritans become too evangelical in their zest for total abstinence, it is as well to remember the wise words of the humorist who said: 'Giving up all alcohol, tobacco and [safer] sex will not necessarily make you live longer—it will just feel like it!'

Persons with HIV or AIDS who have a dependence on 'hard' drugs, such as heroin or cocaine, should ensure that they receive regular advice and support to enable them to withdraw. The use of such drugs

Table 4.2 Choosing food for a healthy life (Courtesy St. Mary's Hospital Nutrition and Dietetic Department)

Healthy eating means eating the right foods in the right balance and the right amount. Food provides you with *energy, protein, vitamins and minerals.*

What are the best foods to choose?

Protein foods Protein plays an important part in the growth and repair of body tissues. Protein foods are: meat, fish, eggs, cheese, milk, pulses (e.g. kidney and haricot beans) and nuts. These foods also provide you with a valuable source of iron, especially red meat and offal. Iron is needed for healthy blood. Milk and dairy products are also good sources of calcium, which is needed for growing bones and teeth.

Vegetables and fruit These foods provide vitamins, particularly vitamin C, for vitality and to keep body tissues in good repair. They also include many minerals. Buy fruit and vegetables fresh whenever possible, but frozen vegetables do provide a good alternative.

Dietary fibre is also present in many vegetables, including frozen and canned peas and beans, and in fruit.

Fats and oils Oil, margarine, butter, lard, etc. These foods are high in calories. Butter and margarine provide vitamins A and D. 'Hidden fats' are also found in chocolate, crisps and salad dressings.

Starchy foods Bread, cereals, potatoes, rice, pasta, breakfast cereals, etc. These foods provide energy, iron, calcium, protein and B vitamins. They are also a very good source of *dietary fibre* and you should aim to:

USE THESE FOODS	INSTEAD OF
Wholemeal flour	White flour
Wholemeal bread	White bread
Wholegrain breakfast cereals—	
e.g. All bran, Bran flakes,	Cornflakes, Rice Krispies,
Shredded Wheat, Weetabix	Frosties
Wholegrain biscuits—e.g.	
Digestive, Ryvita, Bran	
Crispbread	Rich Tea, Cream Crackers
Wholemeal pasta	White pasta
Brown rice	White rice

Beans and pulses are also a very good source of dietary fibre.

Liquid Aim to drink plenty of liquid each day, especially water. It is essential for all body functions.

is a serious medical matter quite independent of (although relevant to) the issue of living with HIV and AIDS, and therefore requires serious medical attention.

Enjoy Yourself!

It may sound trite and misplaced, but hundreds of people with AIDS and HIV have affirmed that their circumstances do not mean the 'end of the world' for them. Many of these persons admit that it took some time for them to appreciate that they did have choices still about the conduct and style of their lives. However, once they came to terms with their diagnosis or positive antibody status, it was as though their lives were starting afresh, with new rules and new goals. They have taken this challenge to heart. One group member described this process as 'learning to put one's self first'.

An impressive aspect of such people is their capacity for enjoyment. Part of the decision to take conscious control of their lives (including discussion with medical staff about which drugs, etc., they may be advised to take) seems to involve a new determination to do some things for fun or pleasure. In a busy life with many demands on time and energy, one may perhaps be required to reassess the reasons for worrying, acting and reacting to the clutter of responsibilities we seem to accumulate. That reassessment can involve *making time for pleasure*. In this busy modern world, it is not always wise to rely on the spontaneous appearance of pleasurable events. Some planning ahead is often required. I think it is best to make this planning for pleasure a habit. There should be a special period each day or week in which personal indulgence is definitely encouraged and expected. The good thing about making time for pleasure is that it does become rather addictive! It doesn't matter what you do—doing it is the important thing.

FINANCE

Financial issues form a major worry for the person with HIV infection and/or disease. There are direct issues, such as the difficulties that will arise if knowledge of infection or the impact of disease results in being excluded from regular work (and thus a regular income). Eligibility for State benefits, and for any action which one may wish to take against one's employer, can be fairly easily sorted out by the relevant authorities. The Terrence Higgins Trust has published an excellent booklet entitled *AIDS and HTLV-III—Social Security and Other Benefits*, which is indispensable for those considering applying for different forms of financial assistance. As for issues relating to one's rights to continued employment and to medical or conventional pensions, it may be worth while approaching either your union (if you belong to one), your solicitor or your local Citizens' Advice Bureau for assistance.

There are also indirect issues of the subsequent status of the seropositive person regarding life insurance, mortgage policies and even retirement or pension benefits. Generally speaking, any such policies taken out before personal knowledge of HIV infection should be respected by the company providing them. If, however, life insurance and endowment mortgage policies are obtained by persons not disclosing their true antibody status at the time they were drawn up, they will be contested by the company when payouts are due or requested.

Getting back to paying the bills: Some people have considered pretty drastic fund-raising measures, such as selling their homes and/or cars. They may do this in order to avoid future worries about paying bills, or to help them in settling debts that cannot otherwise be squared (e.g. because they can no longer work), but any such major decision should be thought over for many weeks before being actioned. Remember how health can influence one's mood!

5
Psychological Adjustments

UNCERTAINTY

The uncertainty relates purely to health. For him it's how long he's going to live. For me, it's how long I am going to have to nurse an invalid. My lover might be ill for six months or a year or more. You can't make any plans for the future. It makes you examine exactly why you stay together. The real point is, is it all going to be worth it? Would I not be better saying now that I'm going to get on with my life now?

Uncertainty about the future is always there, but each day I am certain that I am alive, well and happy. As these days continue the uncertainty diminishes. I plan now for the future and look forward to the day when I can look back on this period of my life.

When I was diagnosed with AIDS, I felt peculiarly relieved. At last I knew what was wrong with me after months of trying to convince my doctor that I was unwell and that something was wrong. I didn't like the diagnosis one bit, but at least now I know where I stand.

What's going to happen now? I've got this virus hanging over me like a ton of bricks about to drop. I feel as though I can't have any more relationships, no kids [and] no one's going to want to employ me. How can I get involved [with anyone] with all this going on? Who says I won't be one of the 10 per cent or whatever that eventually get AIDS?

For most seropositives, uncertainty is possibly the most difficult aspect of infection or disease to manage. In talking to many people about this, I have described uncertainty as being rather like a cloud hanging over the head—it's always there, casting a shadow over everything that's planned and done. The secret is to be able to make the cloud smaller, more manageable, and then put it out of the way. Uncertainty can never be erased altogether, but it can be put in a less intrusive place. Coming to terms with an uncertain future is really what this book is about—finding ways of coping and living with doubt and concern, both your own and that of your carers.

Perhaps it is important to realise that we all live with a level of uncertainty about our lives (and deaths). Yet it is probably true to say that we usually take life for granted unless death comes to close family or friends—'It'll never happen to me' is an oft-repeated phrase. This means that we respond to life-threatening events with a greater degree of shock or trauma than if we were, say, seasoned soldiers or primitive warriors. The 'keep fit' and 'youth' cultures of the 1980s have dulled our acquaintance with personal disease and illness, and the longevity arising from improvements in medical services has distanced us from the realities of death. Physical suffering and despair are phenomena we associate more with the Third World nowadays.

In the context of this book, uncertainty can be described on two general levels. The first concerns the uncertainty felt by seropositives over whether they will develop disease related to their infection sometime in the future, and whether they can do something to avoid this. The second level concerns the progress of disease once it has been diagnosed. The quotes above from seropositives both with and without disease reflect these levels. Many questions can be answered about them, but despite the regular progress of medical understanding, many answers involve some guesswork and few can be answered definitively (e.g. 'How long do I have to wait for a cure?'). In view of this, it is easy to see how anxiety and a sense of hopelessness can grow to a point at which they become overwhelming. It is also easy to see how any media coverage of even the remotest glimmer of hope found in a 'new' drug can lead to an almost hysterical clamouring for information and access to it.

At the time of receiving a diagnosis or a positive antibody test result, much uncertainty can also be seen concerning the reaction of the world around the patient to his or her 'new' HIV-related status. Many people have said that they fear the response of others to them as much as the possible consequences of their infection or disease—this fear can create just as much misery and psychological distress as the infection itself, particularly if they know that their employers/colleagues/friends/lover are negative in their views concerning AIDS and HIV.

The uncertainty felt by patients is also felt by their carers and by the health staff looking after them. Many studies of carers of the chronically ill have shown that carers actually have higher rates of depression and anxiety than the people they are caring for. The reason is that they also suffer the disease, only they do not actually have it. Yet they undergo the same degree of personal revolution in coming to live with it, perhaps with the additional burden of worry about the possibility of their own infection or disease. People with chronic HIV disease but not AIDS have reliably been shown in American studies to have far higher rates of psychological and psychiatric distress than those actually diagnosed as having AIDS: the reason is the greater level of uncertainty about their future.

Doctors and health staff also suffer from the uncertainty of their patients' condition. They desperately want to reassure patients that they will stay well and that a cure will be found, and become equally frustrated when particular treatments don't work or relapses occur. 'Burnout' among health staff managing HIV-related patients is probably due as much to the frustration, stress and despair that currently goes with the job as to the hard work and relatively difficult working conditions many have to work in. One recent study among doctors on the west coast of the United States working in AIDS showed high levels of depression, anxiety, burnout and fears for personal health. This was particularly the case if they spent more than 40 per cent of their time working with people with AIDS (most now spend all their time working with HIV-related disease).

Fighting Uncertainty

There is an excellent American television advertisement that says: 'Fight fear of AIDS with the facts'. The same may be said of fighting uncertainty. Although all your questions cannot be answered effectively with the current level of medical knowledge, some important questions can. Arm yourself with as many facts as you can handle. You have a right to know what your future holds with respect to management and treatment options, so find out. This applies equally to patients and carers. If you want to have some idea of how people have managed with AIDS or HIV infection, there are plenty to choose from! Arrange a visit to the local community agency dealing with AIDS—meet people who have learned to live with their condition and who may be able to offer advice about ways of coping emotionally, financially and otherwise.

The need to keep communicating within a relationship is also important. Some couples stop talking about AIDS or HIV because they feel that they have exhausted the topic, or because they may be afraid of upsetting the other, or perhaps because they don't want to dwell on the subject. But many people may still need to talk with their loved one and will gain much confidence from doing so, despite any repetition that may occur. Remember: uncertainty undermines confidence (like so many of the psychological issues arising from HIV infection and disease). Confidence is a crucial element in learning to master your circumstances, including confidence in your lover/ spouse, friends and family. Talking regularly is a way of demonstrating and giving confidence (once you have mastered what facts there are available).

The clinical consequences of uncertainty—depression, anxiety, and so on—and ways of managing these are discussed further below. With all these issues it is important to remember that you are only human— you will not get on top of it all in a day. Thus, keep a sense of history, and look to your past and present resources on all fronts to help keep future uncertainty to a minimum.

ANXIETY AND STRESS

Anxiety and stress for those with HIV and/or AIDS is unavoidable. The stresses facing anyone in a life-threatening situation are numerous and often very complex. They needn't arise simply from the way persons feel about their health: other people will sometimes contribute to or generate stress by the nature of their own reactions. We have, for example, already seen how fear and rejection can add immeasurably to the practical, physical and emotional burdens of identified seropositives. People with AIDS and HIV who were asked about their anxieties listed the following issues:

- The risk of infection which they presented to others and which others presented to them.

- Social, occupational, domestic and sexual hostility and rejection.

- Being abandoned and left alone in pain.

- An inability to alter their circumstances.

- How to make sure of the best possible physical health in the future.

- The possible appearance of repeated or new infections.

- The ability of their lover/partner/family/friends to cope with their problems.

- The outcome of their infection/disease in the short and long term.

- The availability of appropriate medical and/or dental treatment.

- Being identified as homosexual or a drug user.

- The possible loss of privacy and confidentiality.

● Their future social and sexual (un)acceptability.

● A declining ability to cope in the future.

● The loss of physical and financial independence.

With so many worries arising in the context of diagnosis or a positive antibody result, it is not surprising that sometimes overwhelming physical and emotional reactions result. The important thing about anxiety reactions is that they can mislead the sufferer into thinking that he or she is becoming much worse physically as a result of the infection, when it is actually anxiety that provides the complications. It is useful in the first instance to consider the symptoms that often accompany acute anxiety.

Symptoms of Anxiety

In a state of anxiety, normal behaviour is disrupted in one or more of the following ways:

1. *Agitation and nervousness*   Feeling 'uptight', edgy and restless.
2. *Considerable worry*   Sometimes focusing on precise events or issues, sometimes having vague, drifting anxieties that are difficult to pin down.
3. *Physical symptoms*

      Muscle tension, creating chest pains, neck and back aches, headaches, shaking and tremor, 'knotted' stomach.

      Bowel and bladder agitation, resulting in sporadic or frequent trips to the lavatory.

      Nausea and sometimes vomiting, and difficulties digesting food, sometimes resulting in some weight loss.

      Increased sweating.

      Heart palpitations and 'pounding'.

      Dizziness, light-headedness, and possibly tingling hands and feet.

      Some blurring or 'dulling' of vision.

      Increased sensitivity to noise, temperature, touch and bright light.

      Skin flushes, blemishes and/or rashes.

      A feeling of breathlessness.

      Dry mouth.

      Raised lymph glands (with chronic anxiety).

4. *Sleep difficulties*   Problems in falling asleep, waking early and having more disturbed sleep (perhaps including nightmares).
5. *Physical fatigue*   Loss of stamina and frequent lethargy, with sometimes long periods of a lack of energy.
6. *Cognitive difficulties*   Problems with concentrating, remembering and taking information in; easy distractability and confusion, even with seemingly simple tasks.
7. *Mood changes*   Sudden or rapid changes in mood, sometimes from one extreme to another—e.g. laughter to tears. Some people become uncharacteristically irritable and difficult to communicate with, perhaps becoming snappy and especially demanding with loved ones.
8. *Loss of sexual drive*   A temporary loss of sexual desire or functioning.

Panic Attacks

The longer a person endures a higher than normal level of anxiety, the more vulnerable he or she becomes to the more frequent appearance of symptoms. The severity of symptoms experienced may also increase; and tasks undertaken at work, in the home and socially become harder and less appealing, and take progressively longer to complete. In some cases, where anxiety is a chronic feature (has been endured for some time at a high level), episodes of acute anxiety will occur in sudden, overwhelming 'waves', featuring the physical symptoms mentioned to an extreme degree, along with much alarm and panic at what is happening ('I'm cracking up; I'm going to pass out or have a heart attack and die!'). These episodes are called 'panic attacks', and because they can be so physically involving, they leave the person afterwards feeling very tired emotionally, mentally and physically. Panic attacks can last from a few minutes to a couple of hours. Although they are very distressing to experience, they will not cause serious physical damage. However, because they are so upsetting, the anxious person may fear the possibility of their occurring again so much that he or she will avoid situations in which they may occur, most typically situations outside the home or hospital. Thus, many very anxious people become gradually house-bound or even bed-bound.

It is important to remember that for many persons who have recently become aware of their HIV status, anxiety is not a new event. Many people already suffer habitual anxiety and stress, perhaps from early on in life. They will be accustomed to reacting to life pressures as though they were minor catastrophes, and may have focused on perhaps one or two physical anxiety features or symptoms as being typical of their constant 'state of nerves'—e.g. palpitations, sweating or mild diarrhoea. For all cases, in fact, it is rare to see people complaining of the full range of symptoms presented, although it is not so rare for people to become even more concerned about their condition when the physical symptoms (e.g. gross physical tremor) or perhaps other cognitive features, such as memory and distraction problems, start to interfere with their work.

The range of symptoms that accompany high anxiety have particular importance in the fear-laden context of HIV, simply because of the similarity they have to symptoms of HIV disease such as diarrhoea, nausea, sweating, weight loss, fatigue and skin rashes. Not surprisingly, many persons who mistakenly think that they are infected, and many who are HIV seropositive, interpret these symptoms as signs that their health is declining: their worst fears—that they are on the 'slippery slope' towards AIDS—are 'confirmed'. The anxiety symptoms will frequently then become worse, adding yet further 'confirmation' to their worries. This cycle has been referred to elsewhere as 'pseudo-AIDS'. It is seen most commonly in the 'worried well' and has led in some cases to a suicidal despair. It is, therefore, important for the symptoms and process of anxiety to be well understood, so that people are not encouraged to misinterpret a perfectly understandable—and, to some degree, expected—spectrum of physical and behavioural reactions.

Maintaining Anxiety

The process of anxiety can be thought of as the development of a habit. The habit is sparked off by a traumatic event (such as an AIDS-related diagnosis), which generates the symptoms we have discussed above, and is essentially maintained by the conversations we have with ourselves about that event and the symptoms arising. For example, the person who is aware of the HIV epidemic and the possible risk of exposure to infection might begin by having such thoughts as 'I'm sure I've picked this infection up. How on earth will I cope?' The appearance of lymphadenopathy and a positive antibody result in our hypothetical example lead to further confidence-shattering thoughts ('My God! I'm getting sicker. This is it—I'm going to die') and worsening symptoms of anxiety. Mental images of friends who have developed HIV disease, or even of pictures of ill people in newspapers and on television, become the 'standards' by which our imaginary patient assesses his own likely outcome. These images 'spark off' renewed periods of more intense anxiety symptoms. Memories of the way in which he was unable to manage successfully with the decline and deaths of family members and close friends come to characterise his view of his ability to cope now—in short, he convinces himself that there is only one conceivable outcome of his current infection, and that he will not be able to cope with living with his infection. He has 'made his mind up'. This view of his present and future then dominates his response to illness, and the somatic (physical) effects of his anxieties increase, compounding his health worries.

This scenario is very common in the patients I and my colleagues have seen over the last 3–4 years. One point, however, that seems rarely to receive any acknowledgement is that such a reaction is surely *normal*. Who wouldn't be suffering some form of anxiety in such circumstances? Indeed, it is the case that some degree of anxiety or stress is even desirable in our daily lives—it helps us to keep 'on our toes' during periods of short-lived adversity. In such cases overdiagnosing or overprescribing is detrimental, as it formalises an expected response to adversity that is quite understandable and normal. But, of course, in this context we are talking about anxieties that persist and become counterproductive.

Persistent anxieties lead to a higher than normal or undesirable state of stress. Many researchers have concluded that chronic stress is harmful, both physically *and* immunologically. Reports concerning the stress of bereavement on middle-aged widowers have shown that they suffer higher rates of disease and even mortality in the first year of their bereavement than men of the same age who are not similarly suffering (it seems that people really do die of broken hearts). Work with animals other than man has repeatedly shown that high levels of chronic stress lead to higher rates of cancer or cancer progression. My personal view from observing many hundreds of patients in the context of HIV disease is that psychological factors, including people's vulnerability to stress and anxiety, and their abilities to manage these factors, play an important role in determining the physical response to infection and the likelihood of developing AIDS. Support for this view is seen in many research studies currently under way or nearing completion in the United States, and the same issue is currently being researched in England. There are also parallel findings in research on patients with other chronic diseases, such as cancer.

Overcoming Stress and Anxiety

The major question thus becomes: 'What can I do about overcoming my stress and anxieties?' Well, the answer comes in two stages. The first stage is to recognise that there is indeed a problem with anxiety, to accept that it cannot just be wished away, and that recognition of the problem does not lead on its own to recovery. The habit of anxiety and stress is a hard one to break. Many doctors working in the field of AIDS and HIV have found this out for themselves: one recent study found that medical staff had markedly higher rates of depression, anxiety and stress as a result of their work, particularly if they themselves also belonged to a group at risk for HIV infection. Perhaps the most interesting aspect of this research concerned the finding that higher stress was associated not with the number of years spent working on the problem, but rather with the concentration or intensity of their involvement with it. The significance of this finding for patients is discussed below.

Confidence

Perhaps a reason for recognition not leading automatically to recovery lies in the effects that chronic anxiety can have on *confidence*. Persons who know themselves to be potentially vulnerable to HIV disease will be feeling cautious enough, usually, about exposing themselves to the big bad world. The presence of constant or even episodic extra symptoms associated with worry and fear will often make them even more so. Confidence in their ability to work, to plan ahead for holidays, parties, evenings at the cinema, or even to be with old friends, without some degree of anxious 'collapse' will often be eroded to a very low level. There may be a presiding fear that when they step outside on their own they will 'have a fit' or 'make a scene' by having another panic attack. This general lack of confidence in their ability to cope with anxiety symptoms will sometimes come to characterise their whole view of themselves, as though the coping, life-experienced mature adult that they used to be never actually existed before!

This problem can often be made even more difficult if other means have been adopted in an attempt to hide their symptoms or to summon sufficient 'Dutch courage'—most particularly, alcohol or drugs. Some people may start drinking in an effort to sleep through their stress at night; others may start in order to find some form of release or relaxation. The bad news is that alcohol dependence and drug dependence (prescription and recreational) just make matters worse in the long run, because the background problem of anxiety is not solved. Instead, the anxious person is left with two or three problems on top of the infection, instead of just anxiety.

Another reason for accepting that anxiety and stress is a hard habit to break lies in the mechanism of stress itself. Anxiety, and particularly a panic attack, involves the major organs in the autonomic nervous system (ANS), such as the muscles, heart, lungs, bladder, bowels and sweat glands. If an immediate danger appears or comes to mind (e.g. being told that you have AIDS), adrenaline is released and these and other organs work faster, placing the body in a state of preparation to 'fight or flee'. This is a very primitive and powerful response—if it happens once, it is likely that it will happen again in similar circumstances (e.g. when memories are evoked of the time of diagnosis, or when the diagnosis and its possible implications are considered at other times). Technically speaking, our everyday level of preparedness to deal with stresses can be termed our level of 'baseline arousal'. When many stresses are encountered or the same stress is repeatedly experienced, our level of baseline arousal is gradually increased. Chronically stressed or anxious people have much higher baseline arousal than those who are more generally relaxed, and it is the intensity of this high-stress impact, and its duration, that result often in higher than normal levels of disease and cancer among the sufferers. The problem with chronic high arousal is that the body becomes accustomed to working at this higher level. It takes a long time for the body to work at these higher levels, and, unfortunately, it takes just as long for the body to 'learn' to work at lower, more 'normal', levels. And in order for the body to learn to 'calm down', other factors must be brought to bear on its functioning—in particular, the way persons think about their situation, and the way they behave in their environment.

The second stage in answering the question 'How do I overcome my stresses and anxieties?' lies in recognising that it is unrealistic to think that life with AIDS and HIV can be lived without periods of considerable anxiety, stress and pressure. Of course, there will be times when the stress is unavoidable, the anxieties will seem overwhelming, and the pressures they create will seem intolerable. Because many stresses and anxieties cannot be avoided, they should instead be faced: The best (and most realistic) response is to *learn how to manage these stresses and the situations that give rise to them*.

In learning to manage stress effectively and the anxieties that give rise to maintained periods of stress, it may be helpful to work through the following steps.

Ventilation

For many people, the stress of their condition is made worse by having to 'bottle up' the worries and anxieties that it causes. This may work for a while, but if there is no or little opportunity to let the worries out by simply talking to trusted friends, one can gradually develop a habit of 'smiling depression' or 'cheerful terror'. Many patients have spoken of the fatigue caused by keeping up the appearance of coping (or even that nothing whatever is wrong), yet wobbling perilously on the inside. There is nothing quite so effective at producing a terrible loneliness and depressive despair.

Many people might worry that if they let the facade down, and expose or ventilate their anxieties to someone, they run the risk of collapsing altogether—they fear that their worry is like a bubbling pool of black lava that will erupt from the mountain of their troubles and overwhelm them forever. This is almost never the case. In fact, the reverse is more often true—not letting the steam and lava out will often result in an unpredictable eruption of destructive quality, swamping themselves and any others who might happen to be in the way.

So, make a time for a good, long talk with a close, trusted friend or your counsellor, and put the cards on the table. Discuss your worries, anxieties and fears without trying to explain or justify them—just let it all out. Cry if you want to—it often helps. The main thing is to experience the relief of knowing that someone else knows and understands what the problems are and is prepared to help you sort them out. The next stage is to identify, if you can, from the process of ventilation those particular issues that cause you to grieve and fester in the first place.

Identify the Stresses

Discussing the worries that conspire to make life miserable or difficult should help in identifying particular stresses that maintain the problem. In identifying stresses, it is important to include all those things that give rise to worry. Do not be concerned that some things may sound 'silly' or 'trivial'—if they make you feel bad, then they are not trivial. Some examples might include the way particular people talk to you about your infection or illness; concern over the way a family member is going to react to realising you are gay, or a drug user, or infected with HIV; concern over the effects (if any) of a particular experimental drug regimen; frustration over work matters; physical features associated with anxiety; loss of sexual drive or inclination; problems over housing or paying the bills; and so on. Once you have the worries written down, they become more manageable, and you can embark on the next step. For those worries associated directly with your medical condition, you will be armed with relevant questions that you can ask your doctor when you see him or her again—don't worry if you've asked them already before, the doctor will not be bothered about reminding you of essential personal medical information.

Identify Reasons Why Stresses Exist

It is surprising how many stresses are tolerated without being understood or subjected to change. Work is a classic example. Many people in the People with AIDS Group have expressed surprise at how anxiety- and stress-producing their jobs are or have been without their realising it; only when they have been forced (through the circumstances of their illness) to analyse the causes of their stress have they appreciated that much was due to the accepted and unchallenged routine of unenjoyed daily labour! The same may well be true for most workers; yet, apart from the typical cliché comments about Monday mornings and Friday evenings that we all make, little effort is made to try to change our work patterns and stresses.

For persons wanting to make life less anxious and stressed, it is necessary to adopt a critical stance over their daily routine *and* the exceptional events that may also be a part of their lives. This means identifying the stresses and the reasons for them. Reasons may not always be clear, and it is, therefore, helpful to break stress elements down into major life areas—e.g.:

Love life.
Home life.
Work life.
Leisure life.
Health.
Family life.

Once the major areas have been decided (and there may be more than those in the short list above), break them down further into activities, desires, needs and personnel concerned with each. For example, some elements may be broken down as follows:

● *Love life* Casual sex partners—involving strangers; regular sex—involving lover; prefer anal intercourse—all partners.

● *Family life* Visit family every three months—mother and father; never discuss homosexuality—father antigay; want to be closer to them—fear their reaction to homosexuality; see sister regularly—accepting of situation.

● *Work life* High-stress job—competitive colleagues; much work fatigue—work long hours; not open about sexuality—boss antigay; not open about illness—colleagues' hysteria about AIDS; problems getting time off work for medical check-ups—attitude of boss and situation unknown.

Such a breakdown will soon highlight potential causes of the stress and anxiety that makes general health adjustment so much more difficult. In areas such as health, where chronic fatigue or a loss of any stamina may be identified as a stress in daily functioning, your doctor or counsellor will be able to confirm reasons or causes of the symptom. In many cases a physical symptom complained of as a significant stress creator will be directly attributable to something like chronic anxiety, or depression (see the symptom lists above). You can make your list of potential causes as general or as detailed as you like or find helpful, so long as you don't go too far—too much introversion or psychological speculation can be counterproductive! The best rule is to keep the analysis practical at this stage.

One extremely practical yet well-hidden reason for stress and anxiety rests in the way we talk to ourselves when facing or even leaving behind difficult situations. Consider the habits of speech that are picked up over a lifetime—the phrases and mannerisms that we use whenever certain situations are encountered. For example, 'Oh, no!', 'Here we go again!', 'I told you so!', etc. The same habits develop in the ways we assess and judge our own actions and the actions of others. Many people will almost always interpret their responses as 'confirming evidence' of their worthlessness, inability to cope or to be successful, even when they or events have gone well. We are all familiar with the perfectionist and self-critical type of person who, when praised for something that he or she has done, says that he or she could have done better, or that someone else deserved to win, or some such comment. In the context of AIDS and/or HIV infection, such tendencies may be expressed in self-talk such as 'This is my fault', 'I deserve to be ill', 'I knew it would be me', 'This proves I'm a failure'. Such self-talk is often not said clearly to one's self—usually it comes to the surface more as a set of imperatives or moral restrainers that imply a judgement in themselves (usually a negative one aimed at ourselves). In the words of an American physician, 'We often talk ourselves into the ground'.

In order to see whether such negative self-talk is a reason for personal stress, it may be helpful to keep a short diary for a couple of weeks. The diary should note the date and time of day that stress-related events occur, the nature of the situation, the level of anxiety felt (rated from 0 = completely relaxed to 10 = totally panicked), and the precise thoughts occurring both during and after the situation. It may be set out as in Table 5.1.

Identify Old Coping Styles and Possible New Solutions

Usually the process of identifying the reasons for stress and anxiety felt in the running of our lives will turn up the ways in which we typically try to manage them (if any). With many sources of anxiety, perhaps the usual coping response is *avoidance*—that is, we refuse to face them or do nothing about them. This results in resentment and stress (and maybe a sense of continuing failure) building up. In particular, the self-destructive habit of festering over difficulties increases stress levels

Table 5.1

Date and time	Description of situation	Anxiety felt (0–10)	Thoughts during	Thoughts after

considerably. Where self-talk maintains one in a rut of frustration, anxiety or stress, some direct affirmative countertalk will be required. Unlike the process of meditation or relaxation (which is described below), it may be very useful to say repeatedly to yourself, 'I am a worth-while and good person', or something similar which undermines the automatic negative thinking that has been discussed. It might be helpful to seek the advice of your counsellor about this—he or she may be in a better or more objective position in which to help you re-evaluate your negative self-talk.

With other, more concrete, sources of anxiety and stress, more practical solutions and adjustments may be possible. For example, problems may be alleviated by changing the nature of work routines, domestic arrangements, and so on. In determining the feasibility of such changes, it will be necessary to assess the impact of possible changes on the lives of others. It may not help to stop work altogether, for example, if it means that your lover or spouse is required to work longer hours or make other major adjustments that will make life too difficult or intolerable—this could alter the nature of your relationship and actually create a new source of stress. Remember, the aim is to reduce stress and make it manageable: to attempt to eliminate stress altogether is probably unrealistic. In general, pre-anxiety coping styles may be very useful, although forgotten because of a loss of confidence. Check them out and reuse them as you find appropriate.

List assets and deficits

Part of the solution-finding process includes making a realistic assessment of what degree of change is possible. In all areas there may well be limiting factors that mean that early changes will have to be smaller than desired, or that, perhaps, some changes will just not be possible. For example, the chronic fatigue that some people feel when suffering PGL, ARC and AIDS might make it difficult to spend more time water-skiing! On the other hand, close scrutiny of available options may reveal some surprises—a little rearrangement of responsibilities may make it possible to spend time doing long-desired things without too much bother. It's worth trying to find out. You may also find that you have resources and options available to you that you hadn't previously considered, such as particular people, places and invitations. For example, your lover, 'buddy', family members and/or friends may be able to help with things that either of you had not previously considered. An instance of this might include the other person calling up particular medical or social services on your behalf, if he or she should have more experience in handling medical or other types of information.

So, the most helpful way in which to define the assets and deficits you bring to each individual aspect of your life is to set out the problem areas and list them against the possible solutions you have already considered. In this way, the most realistic future options will become much clearer.

Having done this, next make a list of priorities for future action— i.e. from needs that are the most pressing, down to those that can wait for a while (remember that it is best to take one step at a time!). Having made the list, get to work—your stress mastery has then begun in earnest. An example of this approach to anxiety and stress management is shown in Table 5.2.

Relaxation and Stress Reduction

So far, the approach to reducing stress and anxiety has looked at steps in managing mostly external stresses. Certainly, by modifying the way we involve ourselves with people and events around us, it is possible to also modify the effects such things have on our physical and mental state. It is just as important, however, to get to work on matters internal as well. For instance, the discussion above mentioned the importance of self-talk in maintaining an anxious perspective on the things that have happened (and will happen in the future). How you speak to yourself will largely determine the way you present yourself to others. If you come across to colleagues and friends as someone who thinks himself unimportant, worthless or a perpetual failure, they will start to relate to you in the same way. This, in turn, will confirm your self-view, and so the cycle is complete—and very hard to break out of. This sort of difficulty is summed up in the phrase of a self-deprecating English novelist, who said of herself, 'Once a fat and spotty schoolkid, *always* a fat and spotty schoolkid'.

Table 5.2 Problem chart for man with PGL

Problems	Links/hypotheses	Possible solutions	Difficulties	Assets
(1) Meets all partners in gay bars—difficult to arrange safer sex	Has not developed other ways of meeting people	Develop alternative social outlets: squash club people at work	Only source of social life; known to many people in bars, who expect sex	Assertive; socially skilled; outgoing; likes squash
(2) Wakes early	Depression linked to (3), (4)	Antidepressants; counselling	Dislikes medication	Will take medication if encouraged; puts advice into practice
(3) Feels depressed	Depression linked to (2), (4)	Antidepressants; counselling	As above	As above
(4) Lack of appetite	Depression linked to (2), (3); direct effect of illness	Antidepressants; counselling; encourage to eat appetising diet	Does not feel worth the effort of cooking	Past interest in cookery
(5) Few friends; meets most friends through sex	Linked to (1)	As (1)	As (1)	As (1)
(6) Would like to tell parents he is gay	Not sure how to approach them; not sure of reaction	Get sister to help; role-play how to approach parents with counsellor	Father frequently comments adversely on homosexuals	Sister knows, and could act as mediator

It is important to tap and make use of personal strengths—not personal problems. And no matter how badly you are feeling at the present time, there is no steadfast law of the universe that says that you must always feel this bad, or this confused, upset, helpless, or whatever. There is always room for positive change. This positive change relates not just to the future, but also to the view one may have cultivated about past events, too. Remember how anxious and depressed people tend to see all things—good or bad—as *adding* to their burdens. Good news can seem troublesome because it is in itself disruptive. People who think this way tend to block off all the good things they have done or been associated with. Past love affairs are remembered for the bad things that they gave rise to, rather than for some of the good things or lessons they created. If you tend to think this way, turn your thinking around. Assemble a list of all the things that you have done that gave you satisfaction, a sense of achievement; that suggested personal ability or strength; that made you laugh. Your self-talk should not be exclusively negative—make room for the positive, too.

Some of my patients have called their achievement list their 'ego-booster'. They take their list—which they have written down on a small pocket-sized card—everywhere they go. When they notice that the old negative thinking is gradually seeping back, out comes the card and the repetition of the times when things did, in fact, go right. Other people have found it useful to have such cards with blunt positive personal messages written on them, such as:

'I am a good person.'
'I am a wonderful person.'
'I can make it through this situation.'
'I know I can do it.'
'It is my life, nobody else's.'
'I love myself.'

Repeating such messages may seem novel and perhaps even embarrassing at first, but they are an important way of emphasising that you have a life of your own that is just as precious, worth-while and meaningful as anyone's. Anything that makes you feel better about yourself and helps you to become master again of your life and circumstances is to be encouraged.

A similar card-based idea to help with anxious moments is the 'flash-card'. As with the others, it should be carried around for consultation when required. However, this card has a list of events, people, melodies, holidays, etc., that have made you laugh or have been associated with very good times and unforgettable memories. They are a boon for snapping out of gloom.

A further and very helpful aide in reducing high levels of stress, and particularly the physical symptoms resulting from chronic anxiety, is *relaxation training*. In keeping with the self-mastery theme running through this book, relaxation training is especially helpful in providing a means of personal control over the appearance of anxiety symptoms, both as they occur and in the future. This is because the more you use a physical relaxation technique the less physically predisposed you will be to the future appearance of panic attacks or acute stress. Relaxation helps to lower your general level of stress and tension, and makes you more resistant to the impact of future stresses, but only if the technique is practised regularly. It doesn't particularly matter which technique you use, although hundred of people have said that the technique presented in Table 5.3 has been very helpful (and enjoyable).

If circumstances dictate that muscle tension and relaxation is difficult or inadvisable, a meditation method, such as in Table 5.3, may be helpful. Again, it is important to make the practice of relaxation, whether physical or cognitive, a habit by doing it daily. Your stress has become habitual—countering it effectively must involve the development of an effective counterhabit.

Table 5.3 Instructions for complete relaxation

When you are ready to begin, choose a quiet room and allow yourself at least thirty minutes of uninterrupted relaxation time. Sit in a comfortable chair that has a headrest, or lie on your back on a bed or on the floor. Sit or lie back so that your arms and legs are extended and all parts of your body are supported. You should not have to use any muscles to support yourself. Let the chair, bed or floor support you. Close your eyes.

Stage 1

The method involves first attending to your breathing. With your eyes closed, notice how your breathing will gently slow down to an easy, steady rate. This is your *natural breathing rhythm*, which speeds up as you encounter daily stresses. The natural breathing rhythm involves no effort on your part—it just happens on its own. In attending to your natural breathing rhythm, you may find it helpful to imagine the sight of your chest rising and falling as you breathe in . . . and out . . . and in . . . and out . . . . Just attend quietly to your natural breathing rhythm for three minutes.

Stage 2

The next stage of the complete relaxation method involves muscular tension and relaxation. Using your natural breathing rhythm as a guide, you will tense, then relax muscle groups throughout your body. You will do this twice for each set of muscles. The important thing to remember is that you always *tense* the muscle group *when breathing in*, and let the tension go (i.e. *relax*) *when breathing out*. So, as you are breathing in, tense the muscle group, making the muscles about three-quarters tight (i.e. about 75 per cent of how tight they could become) without creating pain or cramps. The tension is held for two inhalations, then, as you breathe out, the tension is let go. Let it rush out suddenly as you breathe out, as if you are throwing it out of your body. If any tension seems to be left, breathe that away too on the next outward breath. Remember to *keep breathing naturally while you hold on to the tension*, and to tense only one *specific* muscle group concerned at a time. Here's another tip: as you breathe out while letting the tension go, say the word 'relax' softly to yourself (in your mind) so that relaxing is associated directly with breathing out, and with the word 'relax'. After relaxing the muscle group, notice the difference between tension and relaxation, and how the relaxed muscles feel soft, warm and heavy as you breathe the tension away.

Here is a list of the major muscle groups to be relaxed. Progress through the groups in the given order, tensing-then-relaxing *each group twice* before moving on to the next.

1. *Hands*   Tense your hands by making a fist and squeezing. Relax. Repeat.
2. *Forearms*   Bend your hands at the wrists, pointing your fingers straight up. Relax. Repeat.
3. *Biceps*   Try to touch your shoulders with their respective fists, tightening the biceps (upper arms). Relax. Repeat.
4. *Shoulders*   Bring your shoulders up as if to touch your ears with them. Relax. Repeat.
5. *Forehead*   Raise your eyebrows up as far as they will go. Relax. Repeat.
6. *Face*   Wrinkle your nose and tightly close your eyes. Relax. Repeat.
7. *Lips*   Press your lips together tightly. Relax. Repeat.
8. *Tongue*   Push your tongue into the roof of your mouth. Relax. Repeat.
9. *Neck*   Press your head against the back of the chair or on the pillow. Relax. Repeat.
10. *Chest*   Take a deep breath that stretches your chest muscles. Hold it for five seconds, then let it go. Let your breathing rhythm come back to normal, then repeat the cycle.
11. *Stomach*   Tighten and hold in your stomach muscles by 'sucking' it back against your spine. Hold for five seconds, then relax. Allow breathing to settle down, then repeat.
12. *Back*   Arch your back away from the chair. Relax. Repeat.
13. *Legs and thighs*   Lifting your legs from the chair or bed, tighten the thigh muscles. Relax. Repeat.
14. *Calves and feet*   Curl your toes upwards while tightening the muscles in your lower legs. Relax. Repeat.

As you finish relaxing each muscle area, notice the difference as the tension has been let go, how good it feels to be relaxed and warm and heavy for a change. After completing the muscle-relaxation sequence, feel your whole body lying heavy and relaxed, sinking into your chair or bed. Just keep lying there as your natural breathing rhythm continues effortlessly.

Stage 3

The third stage of complete relaxation involves gently focusing the mind away from the stresses of everyday life, while keeping alert and awake. In other words, this involves relaxing the mind as well as the body. The best way to do this is to decide, before the relaxation session begins, on a favourite image or memory that you can explore for five or ten minutes during this last stage. Many people find the image of lying on a warm, sunny beach very relaxing. If this is your chosen image, use your senses to get the most out of it. Imagine you can hear the sound of the waves gently lapping the shore; the sound made by seagulls flying overhead; the feeling of the warm sun on your skin, of the gentle sea breeze, of your body pressing into the warm sand; the colour of the blue sea dappled by sunlight, of the sand; the shape of clouds passing in the sky; the smell of the fresh sea air; the feeling of calm peace and quiet, and of the well-being that comes with being away from it all, alone and content on your beautiful beach.

Other relaxing images or scenes might be the countryside in spring, with all its own sights, sounds, textures, smells and feelings; a favourite meal; or any holiday memory that is sufficiently powerful and interesting for you to be able to explore and enjoy it for some time. The main thing is for you to explore your chosen image as fully as you can, experiencing its sounds, sights, shapes, temperatures, colours, smells and feelings. Remember, you are relaxed and enjoying yourself, letting all your tensions go as you 'float into' your image.

After you have completed stage 3, keep lying there for a few minutes without making any major movement, then slowly become aware of the sounds in the room, and the feeling of your body pressing down, and then *slowly get up*, without any sudden movements or rush.

Taking Charge Again and Enjoying Yourself

Perhaps the most essential element in overcoming chronic anxiety involves the decision to actually do something about it. As with the other problems that living with AIDS and HIV poses, probably the most crucial first step is to face up to the difficulties and say, 'This is *my* life—I am in charge'. It is important to appreciate that, even in the context of major medical decisions (e.g. about particular treatments), you make the decision, even if it is a decision to place medical management in the hands of your doctor. You may not have much external control over the existence of a nasty virus in your system, but you do have the ability to take charge and accept responsibility for what happens next. I have made it clear elsewhere in this book that taking responsibility from now on is possibly a major factor separating survivors from the rest, and separating those who live effectively and even enjoyably from those who become wretched and miserable.

Every situation you encounter may be seen as an opportunity for you to make decisions, to show yourself that you are in charge. A good friend of mine, who always seems to be relaxed and at relative peace with himself, was asked how he did it. He said that life was too short to waste on unwanted 'hassles', and that whenever he was in a situation that caused slight tingles of apprehension, he would ask himself, 'Do I really want to be here?' The resulting 'Yes' or 'No' was all he needed to determine whether he stayed or left. Rather than making him unpopular, as one might fear, this general approach seemed to win the respect and understanding of his friends and associates, and, of course, created the relaxed person I also respect.

Many people I have seen with HIV and AIDS have initially felt that their medical circumstances would be from now on the centre of their lives, around which all other issues would revolve. Everything, they suggested, would be predicated on their HIV situation, leaving little room for 'simple' pleasures (or even complex ones). This is not true at all. It might be at times if serious illness intrudes, but certainly not all the time. You do have scope for enjoying yourself, although, admittedly, you may have some relearning to do. To make this easier, it is a good idea to keep up at least a minimal social life and to consciously plan for pleasures each day. Being in the company of others is good for you. At the very least, it should help to provide a distraction from the HIV-related routine of worry and morbid distress that many people initially complain of. For some people, joining a group of persons in the same boat may be a useful start—it would at least show you that you are not alone, and that life with HIV or AIDS can still be lived successfully.

A Word about Drugs and Anxiety

Many people who feel the particular physical and cognitive discomforts associated with anxiety will wish to have a prescription of anxiolytic medication, such as Valium, Ativan, Librium, etc. These drugs are very helpful for some people, though not all, and while they may be useful in calming the physical symptoms, they do not always work so well with the mental worry that contributes to stress.

The most helpful way of considering such drugs is to think of them as an option when the going gets very tough. They should not be relied upon as a cure-all in chronic anxiety—perhaps for the first few days they may help to keep conspicuous symptoms in check, but there are very real difficulties arising if they are used for much longer. For one thing, the user will soon develop a tolerance to the initial dose, requiring larger and larger amounts if the initial effects are to continue to be obtained. Second, such drugs have a well-known dependency effect—the user becomes both physically and psychologically 'hooked' on them if they are used over a period of months. This makes withdrawing from the drugs very difficult (often resulting in a reappearance of the types of symptoms for which they were originally taken). Third, using such drugs does not cure the anxiety problem—it simply masks its impact. A further problem with such drugs is that they can impair respiration (breathing)—for this reason, anxiolytics often cannot be given when frightened patients are admitted to hospital with AIDS-related pneumonias.

For these reasons, such drugs should be used as a temporary measure only, perhaps to make relatively normal functioning possible while other self-control methods, such as those described above, are practised and perfected.

A further antianxiety drug that is frequently tempting during the time shortly after diagnosis or positive screening is alcohol. The problems with this drug include its addictive qualities; the fact that it is actually a depressant; and its possible damaging effects if used in high quantities over a period of time. This is not to say by any means that some alcohol should not be taken, but, like most things, it is better used in moderation. HIV can make a very effective job of disrupting one's life without the added problem of excessive drinking!

DEPRESSION

> Sometimes I feel that depression can become more regular and last for longer periods of time and that they can be very intense. Antibiotics can cause depression sometimes.

> Suicide in AIDS patients can occur in very subtle ways. For example, by not eating, staying in bed and not getting dressed, and generally failing to look after yourself and your surroundings.

> Depression is inevitable from time to time and the best thing to do is to get out of it as quickly as possible, because it is destructive to one's self physically, mentally and emotionally.

> After I was diagnosed I had the worst three or four weeks of my life. I woke up in the mornings shaking. I wrote a will. I drank rather too heavily. I started having thoughts about what sort of funeral I wanted. I even prayed to a God I didn't believe existed.

Like stress and anxiety, depression is one of the most common human states. It has been part of the recorded human experience since the time of the ancient Egyptians, and current estimates suggest that between 2 per cent and 15 per cent of adults in any given year are depressed. Most people will admit to having periods of feeling down or blue, but for some this experience becomes more severe and longer-lasting. However, most states of depression are self-limiting, and most people improve spontaneously as the conditions that led to their depression get better or as other factors are brought to bear.

Depression is one of the most common psychological reactions in HIV seropositives, especially in the period after their infection is first detected. As this book shows, there are many reasons why this occurs, but some of the more common reasons reported by patients include:

● The apparent 'inevitability' of physical decline and future ill-health.

● The absence of a cure, which results in a feeling of helplessness and powerlessness.

● The limits that infection and/or disease can place on a person's lifestyle: for example, with reduced physical functioning, reduced social acceptability, occupational restrictions and the limits that infection places on sexual expression.

● Actual or anticipated social, occupational, emotional and/or sexual rejection.

When such issues are seen in the context of the enormous upheaval that knowledge of HIV infection or disease creates, it is easy to imagine why people become depressed—some might say that it is inevitable. However, severe depression can make adjustment to knowledge of infection or disease more difficult or longer to achieve. This in itself is problematic, because, as we have already seen, news of personal infection requires the patient to make important decisions about his or her future conduct, and in some cases these decisions have to be made quickly.

Before considering the ways in which the effects of depression can be overcome or accommodated, it is important to be able to recognise depression and some of its effects. The depressed person undergoes the following types of changes.

1. *Depressed mood* Over 90 per cent of people who are depressed report that they feel sad and downcast, miserable, despondent, hopeless and prone to weeping. Depressed people will often say that their moods change very suddenly, with waves of unstoppable tears suddenly following periods of relative calm (and vice versa). It is often easy to spot persons with a depressed mood—they will often look unhappy, and they

might have a droopy posture, poorer grooming and a lower standard of dress than usual for them. Such outward signs are not always a reliable guide, however, as a number of persons will mask their depression behind a smiling facade—these are known as 'smiling depressives'. On the other hand, some people may be so severely depressed that for them any expression of emotion is quite unlikely and they may report feeling 'empty' or 'barren' of any feeling at all.

2. *A loss of interest or pleasure in previously enjoyed activities* Depressed people will often appear flat and dull, and report being unable to find any interest at all in activities that previously they had found enjoyable or interesting. This includes hobbies or other domestic activities: they may lose interest in eating, in sex, in being with friends and in their work. In fact, many depressives are first 'found' by their work colleagues, who may notice that their normal level of activity has disappeared. This is a particularly serious state for those who are self-employed, as they rely on their own efforts to maintain their standard of living.

3. *Feelings of worthlessness and guilt* Many depressed people will come to dismiss any past achievements or current activities as 'nothing special' and, instead of focusing on those things which they have achieved, they will focus more exclusively on previous mistakes, errors of judgement and 'failures'. Some people may become quite obsessed with things that have gone wrong in the past and may end up blaming themselves for those events, even though they may have had nothing to do with the outcomes. In the context of AIDS, in particular, many people will start to suggest that they 'deserve' their infection or disease and that their current situation is 'evidence' of their original worthlessness and guilt.

4. *Low self-esteem* Associated with the worthlessness and guilt described above is the feeling of being a constant failure, of being unworthy, incompetent and inadequate to deal with the responsibilities that they may have 'misguidedly' taken on over the years. Similarly, such persons will avoid making future business or social contacts, because they may say that they are unworthy or unable to make the best of such opportunities.

5. *Helplessness* People who are depressed might say that they are simply incapable of performing even the most routine daily tasks, such as eating, dressing, looking after themselves, bathing and other domestic chores. Many people respond to depression in different ways, of course, but the person who has had higher expectations of personal performance in the past

may be particularly prone to a sense of helplessness, usually because of unrealistic or perfectionistic tendencies. It is easy to see why a person in this category will often respond to depression with a sense of unremitting doom and gloom, suggesting that nothing can possibly go right in the future. Similarly, previously high personal demands will, in the context of this new feeling of helplessness, reinforce the present sense of guilt and worthlessness.

6. *Suicidal thoughts* People who are depressed for a long time or whose depression may be increasingly severe will often consider suicide as the only possible way out of their current circumstances. It is important to realise that, in the majority of cases, *thoughts of suicide are a common, normal and temporary response to unavoidable life-threatening news*. Lovers, carers or family members should not be unduly alarmed about discussion of suicide or suggestions that perhaps this is the best way out. However, it is important to *take such discussions seriously* and to show that you are doing so. It may be important for carers (and patients) to be aware of the potential for suicide in their loved ones and to make certain contingency arrangements—such as keeping dangerous medicines in a secure place, etc. Suicide is discussed in greater detail below.

7. *Anxiety* As many as 70 per cent of people who are depressed report feeling anxious as well, with the associated physical and mental symptoms that are discussed in the previous section. Such anxiety may be seen in the form of restlessness, agitation, crying, weeping, etc., or it may be seen in the form of the more severe and incapacitating panic attacks. It is sometimes difficult to separate anxiety from true depression, because they do coexist so closely.

8. *Thinking difficulties* People who are depressed often report having increasing problems with concentration and memory, along with an indecisiveness and hesitation in speaking or acting that is quite uncharacteristic of their normal behaviour. Other ways in which depression can change thinking include dwelling on the negative possibilities of future actions, dwelling on self-doubt to the level of obsessive rumination, and thinking more slowly than previously, so that otherwise ordinary or routine mental tasks (such as adding up or trying to think of more than one thing at a time) appear quite impossible or take a very long time.

9. *Obsessions and paranoia* Often, as people become more severely depressed, they may show obsessional preoccupations, sometimes with a 'ritualistic response' (see 'Obsessive

States', below). These are usually associated with the felt hopelessness of their condition and the possibility of the appearance of future infection or disease. Some people may ruminate over images of illness in friends or loved ones. Some severely obsessed people will spend a great part of their day checking their bodies repeatedly for signs of infection, although in the newly diagnosed or identified seropositive person some degree of increased bodily checking and worry over the future of the infection is quite natural and common. The crucial difference between understandable worry and an obsessional condition concerns the ability of the person affected to keep alternatives in mind: the obsessional person is 'overwhelmed' mentally with one type of thought only, whereas the 'reasonable' worrier still has a sense of perspective on the situation and can discuss alternative possibilities with some degree of conviction.

In rare cases depressed people might show signs of paranoia, perhaps blaming other people for their present circumstances and, e.g., suggesting that their condition is the result of some plot to discredit their social group or themselves in particular. This, however, is quite rare (although it is helpful to assume that in most cases some *mild* forms of the conditions described are seen for a short period of time).

10. *Other symptoms*   Along with these classic signs of depression, some people may report that time seems to slow down, that nothing seems to happen quickly enough and that everyone else is too slow. Severe depression may also involve a sense of depersonalisation, in which the severely depressed person will come to feel set apart from reality as though observing it from some distance without becoming involved emotionally.

In addition to these psychological symptoms, depression is also associated with a number of physical symptoms:

11. *Loss of energy*   People who are depressed will often say that they feel 'drained' of energy and continually lethargic and tired, often to the extent that they can't face the normal range of activities that non-depressed people would shrug off as being incidental or minimal in terms of physical or mental exertion. Feeling drained and lethargic will often contribute to a loss of motivation to be involved in activities that would otherwise be rewarding. In other instances people who are depressed become tired very easily, which will only add to their feeling of frustration and inadequacy. It is often difficult to separate the

effects of depression from the physical fatigue sometimes associated with PGL and other forms of HIV disease.

12. *Retardation and agitation*   Depressed people will often say that they feel physically slower or clumsy, and in severe cases they may stop moving altogether, perhaps staring fixedly into space as if in a trance. They will walk slowly, with great effort, and will speak in a monosyllabic monotone.

   When people are also agitated—perhaps when the state of depression is combined with conspicuous anxiety—they may show the range of anxiety-related symptoms discussed above. Additionally, they will be easily distracted, nervous and fidgeting frequently. Where people are agitated without showing it outwardly, they may say that their mind is 'in a constant turmoil', making it difficult for them to concentrate properly or to 'think straight'.

13. *Loss of appetite and weight*   A loss of interest in food is very common in depression—when sufferers do eat, they will describe it as an effort (perhaps mentioning that the food they do consume is 'like cotton-wool—bulky and tasteless'). It is, thus, easy to see why depressed persons will often lose weight. On the other hand, a minority of depressed persons will start bingeing on food (or alcohol), particularly when they are alone. Of course, some people will stuff themselves with food if they have recently lost a lot of weight—they will not necessarily be depressed.

14. *Sleep disturbance*   About 80–90 per cent of those who are depressed describe having problems with sleeping. This category includes those with problems falling asleep, waking (sometimes repeatedly) in midevening and/or early in the morning. Additionally, many depressed persons will say that they do not feel refreshed after sleeping, and this will, of course, add to their general feeling of fatigue and malaise. Other reported sleep disturbances include increased sleepiness and sleeping during the day, and vivid nightmares. Those with sleep disturbances will, not unnaturally, feel increasingly exhausted and vulnerable to the effects of negative thinking, anxiety, etc.

15. *Loss of sex drive*   This is a very common early sign of depression and it may create problems with partners, particularly if they have been used to frequent or regular sexual activity. Of course, a loss of sex drive may lead to further problems regarding self-esteem, and it is important to consider that in any psychological or physical disturbance a loss of sex drive is one of the most common early symptoms. Sex drive will usually return as mood improves. (It is worth mentioning that

both sex drive and some sex functions—such as the ability to become aroused, and to have an erection or orgasm—are very vulnerable to the effects of anxiety, and many newly identified and diagnosed seropositives have reported that their sexual drive and/or functioning have been impaired in the early stages, only to return later.)

16. *Bodily symptoms* Some depressed people will experience changes, other than those already mentioned, in their bodily functioning: they may complain of headaches, neckaches, muscle cramps, a dry mouth, breathlessness, palpitations, indigestion and nausea, low backache, sweating, a fine physical shaking or tremor, bladder and bowel agitation, constipation, blurred vision and rheumatic-type pains. If the person is already suffering some physical pain, depression can make it subjectively worse and seemingly impossible to tolerate.

Depression as a Reaction

It is important to remember that while all persons may experience some of these symptoms, it is very rare for people to experience all of them. If we make the assumption that most people with HIV infection or disease who suffer depression do so directly as a result of knowing of their situation, or as a result of the (in)actions of others who know (friends, family, employers, and so on), then it is useful to see the depression as a reaction. This is an important point, for reactive depression is quite a different matter from the more severe and chronic (and disabling) 'endogenous' depression, which usually occurs in older persons and requires a chemical treatment.

Depression as Withdrawal

Other chapters have mentioned the importance of having clear ideas about why you feel the way you do. Depression in this context may be the result of feeling that the end is nigh; that people on whom you rely for a wage, love, affection and/or support no longer want to know you; that the virus has control of your life and future now; that things can never be the same again. On the other hand, you may be depressed because you do actually lack the physical, financial or other resources to do things that previously gave your life meaning (such as travelling, dancing, working, or whatever). Similarly, depression may result from the confusion and seemingly endless pressures associated with learning to understand your situation—being told that you are seropositive can make you and your circumstances seem very vulnerable and/or unstable—confusion is an expert underminer of confidence and control, and results very quickly (in the vulnerable person) in helplessness and depression.

Understandably, many depressed people find that they simply want to withdraw. In many ways depression is most usefully seen as a kind of *withdrawal*, and if one imagines that the depressed person is someone who is withdrawing both emotionally and physically from the world around him or her, it can be easier to understand. Of course, many people who are facing a life-threatening illness or infection will want to cut themselves off from others, in order either to protect them or to attempt to face their situation without encumbering distractions from other people. This is a common mistake made by depressed people. Where patients try to protect their loved ones by not letting on how they really feel, they may avoid all discussion of the subject of HIV or AIDS and end up much worse off emotionally and psychologically. This is because they have bottled up their fears and anxieties so much that they grow out of proportion to their original significance. In the effort to keep worries hidden, they become such a pressure that a sense of perspective on the circumstances is often in danger of being lost, and recovery (both emotional and perhaps physical) is slowed down dramatically.

Summary of Discussion so Far

To summarise, if we accept that it is really normal, for persons who have been recently told that they are seropositive or have HIV disease, to feel some degree of depression—a reactive depression—the experience of depression takes on a new meaning. Although it is tempting to generalise and say that all persons who learn that they are seropositive become depressed and to treat them accordingly, two further issues must also be considered.

1. In most cases the reaction of depression will subside with time.
2. Symptoms of depression (and anxiety) must be 'teased apart' from symptoms of genuine physical illness, such as the disorientation and fatigue caused by PGL and severe disease. It is important to avoid 'formalising' psychological distress when it may be purely a physical or temporary phenomenon.

In many practical ways depression is also a withdrawal from the environment—which is itself seen as a negatively laden place or set of circumstances. It is natural that we should want to get away—to cut ourselves off—when we are depressed, because everything in the world is seen either as a reminder of the negative pressures that had caused us to feel this way or of our personal inability to master the pressures that it gives rise to.

Another important thing about depression is that increasing evidence suggests that depression may result in altered immune functioning. This altered functioning may not cause problems in the normally healthy person, but for those with immune disease the results could be significant. This has not yet been proved in humans; however, it is a well-known observation that depressed persons are more susceptible to common and irritating ailments (such as coughs, colds and bronchial problems), as well as higher rates of cardiovascular and other more serious disorders. In addition, most depressed people take relatively longer to recover from concurrent diseases or infections and, more importantly, they may lose the will to haul themselves back to a state of relative physical normality. Perhaps just as importantly, depressed persons will lose the motivation to make any effort to get over their problems or to get them in a workable perspective, and this not only prolongs their distress, but also can have considerable practical disadvantages, not least of which is the effect it has on their work and on their carers and loved ones.

Practical Theories about Depression

Three of the most practical theories of depression stress the following features, which are usually central to its appearance:

1. Absence of rewards.
2. Loss of control.
3. Distortions in the way we see things.

Absence of Rewards

This model of depression suggests that depressed people remain depressed because, having withdrawn from those persons and activities in their environment that are rewarding, they receive no rewards and encouragement to keep active, so that the motivation to get involved again is lost. The process of withdrawal is, therefore, sustained, with the depressed person making fewer and fewer responses to the environment which are rewardable.

It is easy to imagine how a sense of futility and personal inadequacy can take over once this downward process begins. For example:

> Bill, a previously lively and enthusiastic man with his own business, became very depressed in the days following being told that he was HIV seropositive (he had no symptoms). He was one of the first people in Europe to be

identified as someone who became exposed after a series of heterosexual contacts with prostitutes. He was thinking of becoming engaged to a woman he had known for many months at the time the news was broken. Following the news, however, he dramatically broke off his association with her without any explanation (fearing that she or her friends might tell others). Similarly, he cut himself off from his own friends and withdrew from his business routine (largely because he was too preoccupied with his infection to be able to concentrate effectively). As his inactivity grew, and his devotion to negative thinking about his future increased, so did his depression. He came increasingly to see himself as a failure, regarding all meaningful future options as being closed to him. Eventually, he became almost completely inactive and withdrawn, requiring hospitalisation as the first step to meaningful recovery. The next step involved gradually encouraging Bill to resume his old contacts and routines. How to explain his absences was discussed and rehearsed patiently with the hospital staff, and, as his confidence grew, he became better able to deal with crises and problems that had been left behind or had later developed. Such a process did not happen overnight—he had developed habits of seeing himself and others which were now obstacles to a flexible and confident world view, but over a period of months he got back to the way he thought he used to be. By placing himself in a position where his worth to others could be reaffirmed—and his abilities to cope effectively—he was able slowly to recover from depression.

Loss of Control

This theory of depression is more formally described as 'learned helplessness'. It suggests that people become depressed when they feel that they have no effect on the process or outcome of events—it focuses on the way people construe the relationship between actions and results. More recent versions of this theory have suggested that depression results from people attributing 'bad' outcomes to their own faults of character, and 'good' outcomes to circumstances out of their own control which have nothing to do with their own actions. Depressive events, therefore, come to further 'indicate' the person's inability to 'do things right' because he or she can not have any influence on the outcome of those events.

In the context of HIV infection, it is easy to see how people become depressed: the virus inside them is 'in charge'; they can exercise no influence over its workings (and their potential destruction). As a result of such perspectives, many HIV seropositives lose all self-esteem and withdraw from future attempts to regain control. Increased depression is the inevitable result.

Distortions in the Way We See Things

This theory of depression considers that people become depressed because they are or become very selective in the way they see things—they always look on the black side of themselves, the world and the future. This selective attention may be due to habits of thought which are virtually 'automatic' whenever the person is faced with a new or slightly challenging situation. For example, in meeting a potential employer, the person may say (or, rather, think) to himself: 'I'm going to make a complete hash of this', or 'Here goes another failure'.

With regard to being seropositive, a person may adopt a new variety of automatic thoughts which exemplify the kind of selective and often moralistic thinking that typifies depression—for example:

'No one will ever want to know me again because of my infection.'
'My friend no longer wants to know me because she didn't call me this week.'
'My lover is miserable because he has to put up with me like this.'
'I got this illness—that proves that I'm worthless and bad.'
'If I didn't have HIV, everything would be perfect.'
'I ought to have been more careful—this proves that I'm useless at everything.'
'There's no point in doing anything anymore—I'm just going to die anyway.'

When such self-statements are examined closely, it is clear why they generate and maintain depression: they leave no room for flexibility; they tend to exemplify extremes; they are too black and white. No human being is ever perfectly happy; no one is ever perfect in all things; we all (continue to) make mistakes; our lives all contain some degree of mess or uncontrollable 'hassle'. But depressed people often 'forget' this; they may develop the view that before HIV everything was simply smelling of roses and nothing ever went wrong or was frustratingly complicated. Further, many depressed seropositives will, once they have learnt of their condition, forget that they were ever able to deal with life crises or problems, that they ever had skills or experience in managing upsetting or challenging situations. Instead, they replace their world-wise experience and coping vocabulary with a new set of imperatives and judgements that virtually *guarantee* depression. For example:

'It is a dire necessity for me to be loved or approved of by every significant person in the community.'
'I should be thoroughly competent, adequate and achieving in all possible respects if I am to be considered worth while.'
'It is awful and catastrophic when all things are not the way I wish them to be.'
'Being infected or ill is an indication of my personal worth and "goodness", and the sicker I am the more worthless I am.'
'I will never really experience pleasure or enjoy myself again because of my infection.'

Armed with self-statements and imperatives like these, the seropositive (whether suffering from any illness or not) interprets every situation according to them. They act as universal qualifiers— nothing occurs without being filtered through this mental net. Who wouldn't be depressed as a result?

Summary

To summarise, each of these theories of depression has some degree of overlap with, and relevance to, the other. All of them emphasise deficits in the self-management of influences (practical and cognitive or mental) maintaining depression, and each considers the consequence of a loss of rewards to the individual. By blending them together one can characterise the depressed person as someone who:

1. Attends selectively to negative events.
2. Selectively considers immediate—rather than long-term—explanations for the actions of others.
3. Is overly stringent in judging self.
4. Attributes responsibility for the outcome of situations inaccurately.
5. Has insufficient self-rewards.
6. Is excessively self-punishing.

What to Do about Depression

The discussion above has indicated that the severity and maintenance of depression is, to a considerable degree, open to self-management. What follows is a general plan for understanding and coping with many of the elements which can create and maintain depression. The strategies suggested do not follow any particular order, although starting with monitoring in some form is probably helpful.

Monitoring

There are two areas to monitor.

First, keep a diary of daily events. This will help to shed light on potentially rewarding situations or accomplishments that the nega-tive-thinker may have missed or not recognised. Even mundane daily chores should be recorded—they are evidence, after all, that you are accomplishing something! Also, by keeping a daily record you can develop a picture of what time there is available to do other things, of patterns of activity that may contribute to depression and of those things left undone that may help restore confidence and motivation in the future.

The second area concerns the automatic and self-critical self-statements that may coincide with any activities or events encoun-tered, and that maintain a sense of hopelessness and worthlessness. This may take quite a bit of careful thought—the fact that such self-destructive thinking is often 'automatic' indicates how subtle it is and how uncritical the thinker has become! In keeping this record, try to discern the *first* thought to enter your head whenever you are faced with a challenging or slightly worrying situation or experi-ence—e.g. when someone telephones, when you see an AIDS-related story in the papers or when you think of your own circumstances. Use a record form like the one shown in Table 5.4 to chart your progress.

Table 5.4   Self-statements record form

Date and time	Situational and other 'triggers'	Automatic thoughts	Emotion before and resulting

You will soon find that certain themes may appear in your automatic thinking. They may take the form of 'awfulising' ('It's just *awful* if I look ill in public'), 'musturbating' ('I *must* always show that I'm coping superbly', 'I *should* not be so unhappy when people are around'), or 'damning/blaming' ('I'm such a *failure* because I'm infected—I *deserve* to be ill'). Other types of unhelpful thinking include these sorts of self-statements:

'My lover doesn't love me because he keeps disagreeing with me.'
'If I were dead then I wouldn't cause such problems for everyone.'
'What's the point in trying when nothing is going to change.'
'It's too late to try to make things better now.'

Challenge Your Thoughts

Having made a record of your thinking for a few days, the next step is to challenge the accuracy of these assumptions and thoughts. Ask yourself, 'What am I telling myself that may be unrealistic?' Attempt to re-evaluate your depressive thinking by testing its accuracy against the possible alternative explanations. Distance yourself from the situations giving rise to the automatic thoughts—as if you were an objective observer seeing what (and who) was happening for the first time—and see whether you can generate some objective alternative thoughts that account for the way events unfolded. For example:

'People are avoiding me because of my infection' (automatic thought).
'People do have their own lives to run in the evenings' (alternative 1).
'People may find it difficult to discuss it with me' (alternative 2).
'I've been a bit difficult to talk to lately' (alternative 3).

Because some of the automatic thinking that maintains depression is based on the perfectionistic and exclusive ('black and white') themes described earlier, you may need to talk about your discoveries with others to see whether your perspective on events is actually reasonable. If it is not, rehearse alternative thoughts and self-talk that you can use in similar situations in future.

Talking

Talking to others is probably one of the most helpful things you can do. Discussion with loved ones or close friends may have fallen into well-worn ruts, and you may feel that it does neither of you any good. However, talking can help release bottled-up tensions, and it may be useful to talk instead (or as a first step) with the hospital or clinic counsellor. An outside view can also restore a sense of objectivity to your own view of things. It won't hurt, anyway. My experience suggests that bringing in a sympathetic third party can break the old mould of depressive or frustrating chat (or get people talking when both have really wanted to but neither knew how to start) and bring people closer at a time when they want and need closeness.

Re-evaluate Goals and Responsibilities

Many depressed people have unrealistic goals which, once they have set them for themselves, virtually guarantee a sense of failure because they are out of reasonable reach (at the present time). Do not look too far ahead—you have enough on your plate just coming to terms with the infection/illness and the immediate issues it presents. Go for more realistic and achievable targets—if necessary, by taking just one day at a time. Even the most able and skilled personal managers know that nothing usually gets achieved overnight—things take some patience, planning and persistence. It's the same with finding targets to work your way out of depression.

In a similar vein, it is important to re-evaluate responsibility for your infection/illness and its management. It could be argued, for example, that while having the infection is no one's fault, and just having it is no measure of your personal worth *per se*, what happens next really is up to you and not the social, medical or community system. You are in charge of your body and what happens to it—everything that results in the way of medical care or social or personal circumstances depends in some measure on your decision-making. Statistics about outcome of disease were developed long before you yourself came on the medical scene—they relate to groups, not individuals like you. The major responsibility for your future rests with you. It is yours—not the virus's or the hospital's or the community's. Of course, part of the process of taking responsibility for your circumstances requires that you become informed about what you have and how it is being managed. To do this you will have to talk to your physicians—they will be happy to tell you what they know. And talking, as we have seen, is a very good extra step in the battle to overcome depression.

Increasing Activities Undertaken

The withdrawal that accompanies depression usually results in little being done by the depressed person. This goes even for dressing, washing and eating. Therefore, it is vitally important to start doing more, even basic, tasks to show yourself (and others who may be worrying about you) what you can do. There is nothing to stop you planning long-term projects, but at this stage it is important to break such objectives down into realistic, attainable sub-tasks which can be achieved in the short term.

Perhaps the best first step is to make a list of outstanding domestic and work tasks. If the list seems to be long, don't worry—just by making one you are on the way to sorting them out. Allocate one or two smaller tasks to be done each day—nothing grand, but enough to get momentum going. With the bigger, more complex tasks on the list, see whether you can break them down into smaller sub-tasks which can be tackled separately. You may need the help of other people to get all the bits working together properly or in the right sequence. And, if there are some hitches, don't lose heart. They don't prove anything other than the fact that hitches sometimes arise!

The point about doing things again is that the more you do, the greater the opportunity you have for feeling better—you open yourself up to more rewards and the satisfaction of knowing that you are doing things again at last.

Plan Your Rewards as Well!

While you are doing the things that need to be done, don't forget that there is room for enjoyment as well! Leisure may seem like a frivolous consideration at the moment, but experience suggests that depressed people often need to learn to enjoy themselves again. So, after doing the laundry, watch a film or some television or listen to some music, or whatever. The important thing is that the habit of doing things is associated with the habit of doing pleasurable things. Again, making a list of the activities you (used to) really enjoy may be a useful start.

One patient with AIDS, Charles, found that walking was an activity he could appreciate and enjoy. He would spend some time each day walking in the areas near his home in the country:

> I came out of my first depression while walking in a particular area near my home. I'm not too sure what happened but a feeling of power to overcome came over me. I have since used that spot to help me at similar times and this, together

with notes I have made of particularly happy thoughts or moments, has given me points to go back to for uplift or renewal.

Get Back to Work

If your health permits (and your employer or customers are in favour), start working again as soon as you can. The routine of work, together with the distraction it usually provides, can be an excellent antidote to the preoccupations with AIDS and HIV that many seropositives have to grapple with. The money helps, too. Remember, it will be important to have the story about your absence well-rehearsed before you return (see Chapter 4).

A Word about Drugs

Many depressed seropositives have mentioned that they spent the first few days or weeks drinking, mainly as a sleep-inducer or 'in order to forget'. The only problems with this strategy are that the problems still remain long after you have woken up again (one patient recently said, 'I drink to drown my sorrows but lately they've learnt to swim'), and one can often wake with a nasty headache! Also, alcohol costs money and too much is hazardous to the health. A further difficulty in trying to fight depression with alcohol is that alcohol is itself a depressant. So much for that! Other recreational drugs may provide better short-term effects but they also are health hazards (remember, you have a compromised immune system). So, the general rule is:

'Take care of yourself—have fun and in moderation.'

Severely depressed people may require a course of antidepressant medication, particularly if they start feeling suicidal or become gripped by obsessional problems (see below). Antidepressant drugs themselves are not to be taken lightly. For example, they should not be taken 'off and on', depending on how you are feeling on particular days. If they are to be effective, they should be taken over a period of months and, when the depression has reliably lifted, they should be withdrawn slowly. With most antidepressants there will be a 'break-in' period of at least three weeks before the effects of the drug are reliably felt. However, most antidepressants have side-effects which are themselves discomforting for the first few weeks (they will usually disappear when the body has learned to 'tolerate' them). For this reason we usually recommend that the prescription of antidepressants be given over a period of increasing dosage so that side-effects are minimised (such side-effects include a dry mouth, visual blurring, a hangover and slight muscle tremor).

The type of antidepressant found most useful in our groups of seropositives is the tricyclic family, some of which are also useful in some cases of anxiety and of obsessional conditions. This family of drugs does have one effect which may be of concern in some cases— they may induce a lowering of the body's white cell count (a condition known as leucopenia). For this reason, if you are prescribed a course of antidepressants, your doctor will want to take monthly blood samples to ensure that no such effect is happening with you.

OBSESSIVE STATES

It is easy to see evidence of an obsessive condition in the context of the AIDS and HIV epidemic—signs of it are visible in the nastier printed media every day. A cynical reader might say that the obsession typically concerns not so much a fear of the infection or its impact on society in general as a voyeuristic and savage preoccupation with the private lives of some prominent citizens. Such obsessional 'coverage' of personal and international tragedy merits nothing other than a dustbin.

Aside from the personally intrusive and destructive character of such 'reporting', ill-informed and/or sensationalist media coverage of the HIV epidemic has a further effect: many people who are either infected or non-infected have developed an obsessional degree of worry about their viral status as a result of this coverage, which encourages the reader to fear the infection, its potential consequences and the risks that are presented to others. One might justifiably refer to the resulting social disease of AFRAIDS. And this is quite apart from the vicious scapegoating of known risk groups which appears also to be encouraged in the reader!

On an individual level, it is important to distinguish between, on the one hand, the degree of concern and worry that the seropositive person, or the person at risk, might experience once he or she has learnt of the (risk of) infection, and, on the other hand, the obsessional states that can arise in people who have been unable to adjust to knowledge of their personal vulnerability. For example, people suffering from an obsessional rumination will experience *involuntary* (non-controllable) thoughts or mental pictures of illness, decline and/ or death over and over again, sometimes with these thoughts 'plaguing' them for many fraught hours without relief. The distress is compounded because nothing seems to take the thoughts or images away—past distractions seem not to work no matter how hard they try to resist their worrying thoughts.

Other forms of obsessive rumination include mental checking, in which, for example, people go over and over their past sexual experiences in often amazing detail, in order to try and determine whether any of their past partners showed any signs of ill-health. Another common form of mental checking involves people trying to work out whether they have done anything accidentally which may have exposed their friends, family or loved ones to the virus (e.g. cutting themselves and shedding blood which may have 'contaminated' others).

It is not surprising that the mental oppression of such involuntary preoccupations can lead to the greatest degrees of frustration, exasperation, distress and misery. Such thoughts can take up all the hours in a day, leaving the sufferer exhausted with anxiety. They can lead to great relationship distress, particularly because no amount of urging, encouragement or effort on the part of the carer seems to distract the obsessive from the thoughts of which they despair. A further difficulty is the coinciding of such states often with severe depression (like so many of the psychological issues discussed in this book and by patients, they usually seem to come in 'clusters' of two or three or more).

Another obsessional state involves the ruminations described above occurring with (or more properly, leading to) *compulsive* activity, such as checking, repeating or counting. Typically, an obsessive-compulsive condition involves involuntary (HIV-related) thoughts creating such anxiety in the person thinking them that compulsive activity occurs in order to reduce that anxiety. For example:

> Mrs D was convinced that she had acquired HIV during a brief affair with a neighbour. She became particularly upset about the possibility whenever she read reports of AIDS in the daily newspaper. Her thoughts on the subject became immune to any attempt at distraction and led to such high levels of distress that the only way she could gain even temporary relief from the anxiety was by stripping naked and examining herself from top to toe in the bedroom mirror. Once she had completed this procedure she would be relieved for an hour or two . . . until the thoughts returned and she would have to start checking again.

A further example:

> Mr K, a young haemophiliac with HIV infection, rapidly

became preoccupied with the possibility of developing AIDS. Newspapers had fed his fears with their scary and pessimistic stories, and although he would try to resist the impact and worry that such fears generated, he simply became worn down by it and would spend hours daily searching his body for signs of Kaposi's Sarcoma or skin lesions caused by other infections. If he was interrupted at any time during his daily examination sessions (which also involved counting all his bodily freckles and moles in case there was one extra), he would have to go back to the beginning and start over.

Many patients have observed that obsessive states or periods occur most frequently when they have the time to think about their circumstances. If they are working in a job that requires mental effort and a reasonable amount of attention (particularly jobs involving contact with people), their obsessions seem to stay in the background and they can enjoy time free of their worrying grip. This is yet another reason for seropositives to keep working (if they have a job at the time they discover their infection or disease) for as long as possible—time to think is time to worry!

For others, however, the force of their obsessions is such that they simply cannot work—their distressing thoughts make it well-nigh impossible to do anything of a creative or complex nature. This kind of effect is not new. When women's magazines ran articles on breast cancer and how to diagnose it in the early 1980s, doctors in many parts of the country received many female patients who were convinced that they had discovered breast cancer in themselves and who had developed obsessional states over the possibility of its future appearance. Similar effects were seen when other diseases received wide coverage in the media, such as Legionnaire's Disease and herpes.

It is important, as always, to remember that some degree of obsessionality is to be expected in the immediate period after receiving a positive HIV antibody result or a diagnosis of HIV-related illness. This obsessional concern will usually abate reasonably well as understanding of the circumstances increases and confidence in personal decision-making and management grows. Where the consequence involves a genuine obsessive state, this will resolve over a period of time, without intervention, in about one-third of cases.

There is another kind of obsessional state which has appeared in the context of HIV—the obsession associated with the drive to find the cure for infection or disease. For example, with some people it may involve slavish devotion to a certain method of emotional purging designed to reduce stress and optimise immunological development.

With others it may involve the tyranny of positive thinking whereby people are 'forcing' themselves to think positively at all costs, regarding any 'lapse' into worry or sadness as a crucial failure (I suspect that some carers have fallen into such a trap). There is also the slavish following of 'anticancer' or 'anti-AIDS' health regimens and diets which can be interpreted as a form of obsessional behaviour. When the dice are loaded by HIV infection, it is easy to imagine why any lapsing from such acquired paths as these can be regarded as crucial and serious—people are, after all, embracing values and activities that they see as potentially life-saving, and they are often desperate for them to work. However, as many 'veterans' have said to me in the past few years, any regimen that does not allow some degree of flexibility or room for relaxation (or even pleasurable 'holidays' from them) is, in itself, probably stressful. We are human beings, not machines, and no one can reasonably be expected to get things absolutely right all the time. Your health choices are designed to do you good—not make you even more restricted and miserable. The bottom line is this: be careful with yourself and your life, *and* allow room for manoeuvre and human vulnerability!

What to Do about Obsessive States

Discuss Your Worries about Physical Symptoms with Your Physician

Many people will have obsessional worries 'sparked off' by the appearance of physical 'symptoms' that they fear are either related to their otherwise asymptomatic infection or indicative of a worsening of their illness. There is no point in wondering about such things—ask your doctor. Given that many people are already in a state of considerable anxiety about their infection, it is quite likely that the sorts of physical changes causing the concern are due to anxiety (symptoms of anxiety are described fully in pages 67–68). A number of research studies conducted overseas have found that the greatest levels of worry and anxiety (and physical symptoms of these) are seen in people with symptoms of HIV infection who do not have AIDS (i.e. they may have PGL and/or what used to be called ARC—now called chronic HIV infection). This finding has been explained by the greater levels of uncertainty felt by such groups—the occurrence of some symptoms of infection generates uncertainty and concern about the possibility of those symptoms becoming worse. People with asymptomatic infection do not have these worrying signs and people with AIDS know more precisely what their enemy is—their uncertainty is more precisely focused.

For most persons, the advice and expertise of their doctor will be sufficient to allay their concerns about the appearance of minor or disturbing physical changes. However, many people will find that this step is of temporary benefit only, and before long they will find themselves back at square one, particularly if they have seen yet another example of media obsessionality since they last saw their doctor or counsellor.

Avoid Media Coverage of AIDS and HIV

Because so much of the distress related to obsessional states is generated by media (mis-)treatment of HIV and AIDS, it seems sensible simply to avoid exposing one's self to such upsetting material. It has, sadly, often been the case that after considerable periods of time spent in building confidence and mastering symptoms of anxiety and stress, people reading gloomy, inaccurate or hysterical coverage have had that confidence and mastery completely undermined. Their despair and frustration has been felt equally by carers also, and some relationships have fallen apart because of the stress caused by re-emerging obsessions.

Practise Past Distractions

In the previous section, on depression, there was a quote from Charles concerning his 'special place' for walking and uplifting his morale whenever he felt low. Similarly, in the section on anxiety (above), mention was made of 'flash-cards' and 'ego-boosters' as ways of diverting one's self away from gloomy or anxiety-producing thoughts. Although the present discussion has emphasised that attempting to distract thinking away from the obsessional thought or image is often futile at the time it appears, it may still be helpful to have some 'counter-ritual' planned for those times when such thoughts are likely to occur. One patient said recently that, as long as he had his day planned carefully, he would usually not be troubled too much by his obsessions, but the important thing for him was always to have something to do or think about instead at the vulnerable times.

In order to have effective contingencies arranged in advance, you will, of course, need to identify clearly what the most vulnerable times are. If you keep a record of the times when the obsessions strike, or go back over the difficult times of the past couple of weeks, they should be pretty clear.

Response Prevention

For those people whose distress at the obsessive ruminations leads them to compulsive checking or other compulsive activities, it may be quite helpful to limit the amount of time given over to physical checking and thereby limit the disruption it causes. This can be done in a number of ways. First, prepare for the vulnerable times in advance, as suggested above. Second, when the compulsive urge appears, resist checking more than once. Make a checklist of those parts of the body that can be scrutinised and tick them off as you have checked them (allowing a specific time, e.g. thirty seconds, for checking each area). Another form of response prevention is to check only once at particular times of the day, reducing the number of daily checks as the days go by. Obvious daily periods for limited checking include times spent bathing and dressing, or undressing prior to bed.

Drug Treatments

For people who have tried such measures and who still remain gripped and severely disadvantaged by their obsessive disorder, a form of antidepressant may be the only remaining possibility. This is particularly so where the person affected is also severely depressed (bearing in mind that many people become obsessed after they have suffered unremitting depression for a time). One type of antidepressant, clomipramine hydrochloride, has been found to be helpful in cases of obsessional disorder, although its effects on this are by no means guaranteed. It is also important to remember the need for careful monitoring of white blood cell levels if such drugs are prescribed, as they may cause leucopenia in some people.

SUICIDE

Suicide in AIDS patients can occur in very subtle ways.

It has been said (by a well-known British novelist) that the only really worth-while subjects of adult conversation are sex and death. Although many people might disagree, it seems pretty clear from conversations with seropositives that sex and death are at least two of the major post-diagnostic subjects of contemplation, particularly where illness is at hand.

It is important to remember that thoughts of suicide are a common and normal response to unavoidable life-threatening news. I have lost track of the numbers of patients who have made, some months after they were told of their infection, such statements as 'I kept thinking that I would kill myself now rather than let the virus do it slowly'— particularly when sensational newspaper headlines appear with an emphasis on death and decay. Speculation and the frenzy for attention-grabbing media statements can turn the life of a seropositive into a world of relentless, morbid gloom in which the option of suicide may come to seem a serene retreat.

It is also important to remember that, at the time of writing, no vaccine or cure for HIV infection has been found or even appears imminent, and speculation has focused on the possibility that *all* HIV seropositives may eventually develop AIDS or dementia as time passes. Many may genuinely feel that the dignity of a self-determined death is far preferable to the prospect of an invidious decline. It is also the experience of many doctors and counsellors working in the field of HIV infection and disease that suicide is a rare phenomenon; as stated elsewhere in this book, people with HIV and AIDS want to *live*!

There are many indications for the potential of suicide in seropositives, and in their (seropositive) loved ones and carers. Studies of the people who have attempted suicide highlight the following issues behind their attempts:

Recent 'marital' separation, divorce or bereavement.
Impending loss of a loved one.
Living alone.
Social isolation.
Financial problems.
Poor physical health.
(Recently) unemployed or retired.
Recent violent relationship quarrels.
Incapacitating uncurable illness.
Depression.
Alcohol and/or drug dependency.
Organic brain syndromes.
Previous suicide attempts (especially violent in last twelve months).
Warnings or talk of suicide.
Preparation of means, suicide notes, making will/insurance plans.

When one considers the number of issues in the above list which are relevant to the often recently turbulent lives of the newly identified or diagnosed seropositive, it may appear surprising that rates of suicide in seropositives are not higher.

Many of the people I have spoken to say that the thoughts of suicide were largely relieved when they were given more information about their circumstances. However, despite vast improvements over the past couple of years in the ways that seropositives are counselled and informed about the meaning of HIV in their lives, it is still not uncommon for many people to be left largely 'in the dark' about their health status and its implications.

Of course, in the period of shock that immediately follows after identification of personal seropositivity, it may be more likely that an impulsive act of suicide occurs, perhaps after a period of heavy drinking. It is clear that a majority of suicidal attempts occur in the context of chronic depression, and it is wise to keep a gentle eye on those who are depressed, precisely for this reason. One person with AIDS has suggested that where depression is a factor, the decreased self-care, inattention to eating and general withdrawal may be a form of 'slow suicide'—a gentle withdrawal from life.

It has already been mentioned that the expression of suicidal ideas is not necessarily an indication of the desire to kill one's self. For many people a discussion of self-determined death is a way of asserting a desire for full personal control over their lives, in the context of the frustration, anger and uncertainty surrounding their infection and/or illness. In her marvellous book called *Facing Death: Patients, Families and Professionals*, Dr Averil Stedeford suggests that in cases of truly depressive suicidal thinking, patients will usually be motivated by feelings of unworthiness and guilt, perhaps suggesting, for example, that they 'deserve' to die because of the difficulties 'they' create for their loved ones.

In other cases, where suicidal ideas are not based simply on a desire to self-destruct, they may reflect the desire not to be a burden or pressure in the lives of their loved ones. Some might bring up talk of suicide as a means of 'testing' the readiness of loved ones and carers to 'stand by' them if the going gets tougher. Such talk reflects the intense personal insecurity that HIV can generate, largely because of its documented social and occupational consequences in a basically young and mobile population. Some people, feeling unsure of the 'full picture' of their situation, may introduce the topic of suicide as a 'test' for carers' 'true perceptions' of their future; bringing such a subject up may be seen as a way of forcing the facts out into the open. Many people with infection and/or disease fear a future of pain, and talk of suicide may reflect a wish to avoid the pain and indignity of future or terminal decline. Many people will develop (often very detailed) contingency plans for suicide if their disease reaches a certain stage, beyond which they will become largely dependent upon others. Making such plans involves a level of self-determination and planning that in itself may help the patient to feel that he or she still has an important degree of personal mastery—whatever happens in the future.

Whatever the real motive behind discussion of suicide, it is crucially important to *take it seriously*. Many health staff have reported that suicide attempts can follow patients' perception that their concerns about dying were dismissed or trivialised, resulting in an impulsive attempt aimed at showing that they do mean business (even when they may not have done so when the subject was first brought up). While taking such talk seriously, stay calm—do not be panicked into hysteria or conspicuous alarm. Such reactions do not help people to feel confident about one's coping abilities or sense of perspective! Take care to understand as much as possible about why the patient (or carer) is talking about his or her own self-inflicted death, and use this information as a basis for constructive counter-talk about appropriate future care and management.

Where plans for suicide in the future are unearthed, it is also important to talk about why they have been made, and to reassure the patient that, despite all care being taken medically to ensure that he or she will not suffer pain or indignity, desires for self-determination will also be respected. When some patients are hospitalised, for instance, they will make clear their desires not to be treated beyond a certain level of disease progression; medical staff will usually respect such wishes after full discussion with the patient and colleagues (they may rightly wish to argue about it if they think that there is a good prospect for recovery from disease episodes!). It is important to consider that medical staff generally now consider not only the disease, but also the person when contemplating major treatment decisions: quality of life is a vital consideration in making the decision about how to treat. There is also the fortunate and increasing recognition of the difference between prolonging life and prolonging death. In the past a number of patients have said that their plans for self-destruction were formulated because they feared that hospital staff might not understand this vital distinction.

It is important also to remember that there exists a wide level of hospital and community expertise to help in managing HIV-related disease and the issues it gives rise to. Where discussion of suicide is serious and urgent, do not be afraid to call on the expertise of others who may have dealt with similar situations—their job is to help.

I have noticed in some sad instances how the carers/lovers of people with AIDS, having witnessed the discomfited decline of their loved one while knowing themselves to be seropositive also, have determined to end their own lives once they themselves have developed disease. Their loved one has for them been a kind of model of coping with AIDS, particularly if he or she has died miserably or in great sadness and despair. Accordingly, they may say to themselves that it will be so for them, and they make a suicidal attempt in order to avoid such a decline. This emphasises the vital need for counselling to be provided to all those who have lost loved ones to the diseases of AIDS, and particularly to those who may themselves also be infected.

A final note: in some countries it is illegal to kill yourself. Doing so also has important financial and social consequences. For example, possible suicides (people who may have died by their own hand) will be discussed in the local coroner's court. There is a possibility that the name of the deceased will be available to the media, who may then present the facts of the court hearing in a way that leads to the identification of lovers, family and friends. In addition, insurance companies will usually not pay out on the life insurance of someone who has 'officially' committed suicide.

Further, doctors are not entitled to kill their patients. Committing suicide on a ward may well implicate ward and hospital staff, and lead to considerable professional 'hassle' and distress (quite apart from the distress they would feel at the loss of any patient they have cared for).

If you are feeling suicidal, it may help to talk again to someone— there is, after all, everything to gain by doing so.

6
Relationship Adjustments

The wide range of psychological issues already discussed in this book have a clear consequence: they change the way that a seropositive person relates to those around him or her. Anxiety, for example, can lead to a clinging overdependence on hospital staff, lovers and/or carers:

> John, a 39-year-old salesman, became very anxious about the possibility of new symptoms of his infection. He became overscrupulous about personal hygiene and would collapse in tears if ever he thought he would be left alone in the house by his partner (who had to work regularly to support them both). In addition, he would not move out of the house alone, demanding that his partner accompany him everywhere and preferably do everything for him. His partner soon became exasperated by John's behaviour, particularly when he would seem to 'break down' completely and start tearfully begging never to be left alone at any time.

Similar scenarios have been described by hospital staff and community volunteers, often including the partner seeking to 'escape' altogether, with predictable consequences for the patient. Staff themselves have described anxious patients who might drop in or telephone daily, often repeating the questions they asked last time or sometimes saying very little at all—they have just wanted the confidence generated by understanding human company. Anxiety also seems to be responsible for a kind of hypochondria, in which every physical nuance is interpreted by the patient as sure evidence of physical deterioration. The obsessive-compulsive states described in Chapter 5 often result.

Anger is a kind of mortar cementing barriers between people—particularly when the anger is displaced (i.e. pushed on to others). Staff may, for example, find themselves on the receiving end of abuse and constant—often nit-picking—criticism. Carers, lovers and close family members may become quite bewildered at the torrents of anger that greet them when they appear, and resentment and anger may then be fed both ways, resulting in broken relationships. It has been necessary, in my experience, to give lovers 'permission' to absent themselves from the patient or the home for some time until the anger dissipates or is resolved by some intervention. It is certainly helpful if all have explained to them that feelings of anger are an expected consequence of the frustration and helplessness that many people feel after learning of their infection or disease, and that it is usually a mistake to take the natural expression of these feelings personally.

Fear, depression, guilt and the other possible reactions to life-threatening news are all powerful and can all change relationships. Examples are seen in those who respond to news of their infection by guiltily assuming that HIV typifies their 'true' worth or value in general, and to others in particular. They wrongly see themselves as 'blameworthy' examples of people whose lives have been bad or sinful, and suffer torment and withdrawal as a result. A further type of interference is that caused by physical and neurological changes and damage. For example, consider the impact of early dementia, or increasing loss of sight, or other central nervous system dysfunctions, on the running and dynamics of a young, vigorous relationship. How prepared are any of us to commit ourselves completely to managing the everyday difficulties faced by someone with bowel and bladder incontinence and diarrhoea, for example? The stresses of such problems on relationships cannot ever be overestimated.

Depression and withdrawal in patients have special significance for carers and loved ones. Spending hours or days with a depressed seropositive can lead to a sense of futility and helplessness. Seeing the presence of the virus in the patient's system as a 'time bomb' just ticking gently away until it explodes into disease—as many people do—is bound to induce a sense of helplessness in those affected, both directly and indirectly. Many carers I have spoken to have said that the lost motivation accompanying depression is one of the hardest things to deal with. All suggestions for having a good time or cheering the loved one up are dismissed, all previous hobbies or interests are rejected—'there is no point anymore'. Counter-arguments seem to have little positive impact, carers say. The final result for many lovers and carers has been an almost desperate need to get away—to escape from the tyranny of despair and the frustration of self-pity. There is also a need to have a break away, from time to time, from the agony of seeing a loved one brought down by illness without a known cure. Studies of the effects of other chronic illnesses on carers have uniformly shown that they suffer higher levels of depression and psychological difficulty than are experienced by patients themselves (including alcoholism, attempted suicide, drug dependence, etc.). It seems clear that where carers fear that they are being drawn into the negativity and despair of the person who is chronically depressed, they should be given 'permission' to take a temporary break away, for the sake of both parties.

The psychological problems experienced by carers for patients with other chronic diseases are certainly seen in many of the couples I have seen in the context of AIDS and HIV. There are probably a number of reasons for this.

For instance, where the diagnosis is being kept hidden from others, for whatever reason, the strain that arises from 'bottling up' the tremendous stress and worry can lead to serious mental and physical consequences.

Emily, a vivacious 39-year-old mother of two, was aware that her husband had not been well for many months, but they both thought that he was just 'run down' with the pressures caused by his job as a salesman. When he was eventually given a diagnosis of AIDS, she was told straight away. She and her husband agreed to keep the news to themselves— after all, they didn't want their friends to avoid them or their children. Also, being aware that their children might become targets of cruel gossip at school, they decided not to tell them of his illness. Although they coped well together for a couple of weeks (her husband was still comparatively fit and continued to work as he had always done), the worry, together with the increasing tide of pessimistic newspaper and television coverage of the disease, began to take a toll. Emily slept very poorly, lost weight through anxiety and not eating properly, and gradually lost her patience with the children and those she met during the week. Continuing concern about future finances also became an obsession, leading to many arguments and increasing distrust. It was clear that Emily and her husband were heading for a separation that neither wanted. After two months, she finally agreed to join her husband for counselling and treatment of her own difficulties. One of the most important outcomes was that they both agreed that others should be brought in on their circumstances, although they did not want close friends to know exactly what the diagnosis was. After settling on 'leukaemia' as the culprit, they were able to share their distress with trusted friends, who quickly sprang to their aid. They were at least able to talk to others of their anxieties for each other and their children and to organise contingency plans for the future. With time and patience,

Emily began to feel more secure with the relationship. Eventually the children were told that their father was seriously ill, and the family was restored and reunited in their efforts to pull together and enjoy what things they could as a group.

A further common issue that can create severe difficulties for lovers or spouses is the worry that they too might have the infection and fall ill. There are reasonable grounds for such anxiety, as between 9 per cent and 71 per cent of regular sexual partners also develop infection from the infected other if appropriate precautions are not taken during sexual activity. At least two important issues come to mind immediately about this. First, for a female partner, becoming infected is particularly significant if she plans to become pregnant in future (see Chapter 4) or is already so. The need to avoid pregnancy, or to consider termination, is paramount for the sake of both mother and child. For mothers with AIDS, the spectrum of anxieties over the care and welfare of the children both now and in the future requires the most patient and sensitive discussion. This is in addition to the unresolvable concern that may arise over a future life in which pregnancy is effectively a closed option. The second issue concerns the modelling of AIDS illness that occurs in relationships where both partners are known to be infected. In some relationships where one person has chronic disease, the way in which he or she copes can act as a model for the partner if he or she, too, should fall ill. If the first patient has been despondent or not been able to adjust successfully to altered circumstances, such an approach will often be 'mirrored' by the other. In this way, the psychological problems evident in a relationship will be repeated. Happily, however, the same can also apply if the first patient responds successfully.

Further strains may result from the change of role which may occur in a relationship facing AIDS or HIV. The lover/spouse may suddenly find that he or she has to take on the role of domestic manager, in-house psychologist and counsellor, financial provider and entertainer, while the partner lover is facing his or her new role of hospital patient and medical curiosity. Some relationships can not sustain such pressures for very long, and, sadly, a split may occur. In other cases the challenge of a new, hopefully temporary, career is taken up with some degree of success, the problems only arising after the patient returns to previous fitness and there are then two chiefs and no indians!

What such points underscore is that partners (lovers, spouses) suffer HIV infection and/or disease just as much as if not more than the patient, albeit indirectly. Their lives are subject to the same types of revolutionary pressures and upheavals, while they have to wait and hope that they will not also be in the same boat eventually. This waiting constitutes a special kind of uncertainty, the outcome of which is already being modelled for them in a stark and unavoidable way. It is no surprise, therefore, that they, too, should suffer the same psychosocial handicaps as their loved ones. At the same time, they probably suffer more, because at least their loved ones know what their enemy finally is.

A further strain on lovers/spouses is the lack of open and clear communication about the illness or infection which can frequently arise for various reasons. For example, some people won't talk about their illness because they are trying to protect their loved one from unnecessary worry and distress; it might be thought that if HIV is not spoken of, it will remain out of mind and anxiety will cease. Unfortunately, this is almost always wrong! Both sides of the relationship may be bursting for want of open discussion, each fearing the possible effects of doing so on the other.

A further reason for not speaking of the situation with lovers/spouses is that there may be a fear of boring them with constant dwelling on particular issues. Of course, so many worries to do with HIV and AIDS-related illness are unanswerable—e.g. will the condition get worse? And specific issues—e.g. the effects on the children, to work or not to work, etc.—have no hard or fast solution that can be applied to resolve uncertainty. It is not surprising, therefore, that they arise again and again as confidence or health goes up and down.

Furthermore, some people will not talk of their condition simply because they do not know what to say about it. They may be poorly informed, or they may be depressed or too shocked to face the issues that come up. I know of many people who have avoided discussing their illness or infection because talking about it simply upsets them too much. They try to avoid the distress by blocking out all references to it and keeping quiet. And many lovers have done the same for the same reasons. An extension of this situation is seen occasionally in those people who have always been vulnerable psychologically (i.e. had some form of psychological difficulty, such as a chronic anxiety state, depression or difficulty in making lasting relationships), yet managed to keep it 'under wraps' or under control—they could function 'normally' despite their problem. For these people, learning of their HIV infection or disease may 'take the lid off' their background difficulty by making it much worse and much more public. Such persons may have a catastrophic reaction, and any further reminder of their situation in the form of media coverage or discussion and remarks by friends will cause a further emotional eruption. Their extra vulnerability will encourage them and their loved ones to 'clam up' almost completely in order to avoid this extra distress.

Finally, there are those who use their diagnosis or infection as a barrier. This news is (openly or covertly) used as a justification for not allowing others to get close—it may 'help' to maintain an emotional isolation that has always been typical of the patient, keeping away those people who may otherwise 'break through' and expose them to the scary business of being liked or loved.

INVOLVING LOVERS AND SPOUSES

There are very good reasons for avoiding the trap of non-communication about the circumstances of illness or infection and directly involving loved ones (particularly if there is an ongoing sexual relationship).

1. In order to develop a mutual understanding of the adjustments in sexual behaviour guaranteeing that no further infections will be passed on or received (see Chapter 4).
2. In order to develop a mutual understanding of appropriate standards of domestic hygiene (e.g. in the event of domestic accidents involving spillages of bodily fluids—see Chapter 4).
3. In order to clarify any fears that might be lurking about the infectiousness of the patient and the transmissibility of HIV (e.g. through shared utensils, sheets, etc.—see Chapter 4).
4. In order to enable the lover/spouse to be able confidently to answer questions arising from friends and colleagues aware of the patient's status, and to translate the needs of the patient into language these others will understand.
5. In order to supply the loved one with information about the physical, psychological and emotional changes and needs that the patient is experiencing, so they will be familiar and understandable and not open to misinterpretation (see above).
6. In order to help the loved one to become a confident 'at-home' therapist who can give the hospital and community physicians and counsellors vital extra information on how the patient is coping and, at the same time, apply effective ways of managing the difficult times at home. (One of the continuing fears expressed by patients is whether the loved one will be able to cope with them at home—training by the counsellor or physician may make a great difference in enabling the loved one to do just that, thus also helping allay this patient anxiety.)
7. In order to maintain patient motivation to keep up links with

medical facilities and staff. It is a frequent experience that the degree and quality of patient contact is enhanced when loved ones are also a part of the ongoing counselling process.

These are really practical payoffs from the active involvement of lovers and carers, but they do not convey the whole benefit arising. In short, by having a continual agreement to share and exchange information through regular discussion, lovers and spouses can develop a quality of caring and determination in the face of HIV that gives a vital extra strength and dimension to the whole art of effective coping. Charles, a People with AIDS Group veteran, put this point in his own words:

> Those closest to one may tend to try to shield and protect one by not discussing how *they* feel about the situation. My wellbeing has to be balanced by [that of] those around me and it is important that we are all open with each other and face the prospects in a spirit of togetherness.

It is important also to recognise that every relationship has its own pattern and styles of coping and communicating. For example, some observers of partnerships in distress have noticed how closer, more emotionally intense relationships may result in less overt discussion of serious illness and the possible consequences (perhaps because there is a deeper mutual understanding that does not require spoken words; perhaps because there is a greater fear of loss). Other relationships may require a neutral intermediary to help develop and maintain effective discussion about the feelings held within. On the whole, though, the general observation repeated throughout this book—that open communication about the things that matter gives the best results—applies just as much here. Talking helps with the painful process of acceptance, and acceptance is a vital step to achieving the psychological harmony that 'veterans' of HIV infection and disease seem to have in common. This can create interesting results apart from the obvious ones, as John discovered:

> I've fallen in love! Isn't this a paradox of the most peculiar sort—that it was only when I got AIDS that the time was opportune for a *celibate* love affair, or more, for my first long-term relationship to start!?

Many people anxious to avoid the traps of non-communication and of too much communication have asked how to strike the balance. The most practical solution is first to agree that some talking is necessary. The hospital or clinic counsellor, or community group counsellor, might be a good person with whom to get the ball rolling in this respect—they may be able to help with establishing the first important topics of conversation on 'safe' ground. To keep the ball rolling without too much effort, it might be helpful to use a tip from sex therapy—i.e. planning time for serious talk. If both sides know that there is a certain time of the day or times of the week when open talk is allowed, they will both have time to prepare themselves and what they want or need to say. Having special talk-times means that spontaneous AIDS talk is less likely to intrude on the quiet or good times. I call this 'pigeonholing': topics and worries are placed in their own pigeonhole and taken out when the time is right. They don't then hang like a big black cloud over the rest of the day, casting a negative shadow. And there is the guarantee that the pigeonhole will be examined each day for a specific time. It has worked with many people who felt that their bottling up of concern was making matters much worse on both sides. There is one 'but', however: start the talk-times with conventional courtesies. People with HIV disease can get very tired very quickly without apparent warning (even they may not know when this will happen). There should, therefore, be the exploratory question, 'How are you feeling?', or 'How is your energy level?', or 'How long do you feel able to talk for?' before tiring and taxing issues are entered upon. Also, some people may not be ready or feel sufficiently strong for displays of deep emotion, and some judgement will be needed to assess tolerance on both sides for the consequences of straight talking.

Of course, there may be difficult situations in which non-communication results from other imperatives. A common example is that of the person who has acquired HIV through infidelity and is afraid or reluctant to tell his or her regular lover/spouse (a) because he or she might leave, and (b) because he or she can't face the possibility that the lover/spouse, too, may be unwittingly infected. However, the possibility must be faced—particularly in women, who may become pregnant (for reasons given above). The issue of how to encourage patients to tell their partners has been the subject of intense debate in medical circles for the last few years, and opinions often seem irrevocably divided. My view is that as health professionals we have an obligation to inform our patients as best we can about their circumstances, but we do not usually have any further obligation or rights than that (e.g. we do not have a right to tell our patients to do anything or to demand that they do so[*]). In those cases where others (i.e. lovers/spouses) may unwittingly face the risk of infection, it would seem necessary to inform patients of the possible consequences

*In England there is a statute enabling the enforced detention in hospital of HIV seropositive persons who, if allowed out, may constitute a risk to others in the population. It has been used only once, at time of writing.

for the other should they develop disease and/or become pregnant in those situations where stable relationships exist. Where relationships are casual, however, routine advice on safer sex seems appropriate.

Getting back to the main point: in stable relationships there is no other routine advice that can be given to the patient other than the need to give as much information to the lover/spouse as possible. Further, it is, in my experience, usually better for the lover/spouse to be told sooner rather than later.

FRIENDS AND FAMILIES

All persons and all families have their own way of coping with the impact of HIV infection and/or disease. However, where the facts are not known or understood, some degree of misunderstanding or rejection of the patient is probably inevitable. The fear of rejection is probably the greatest single reason given by patients for not informing their friends and family of their illness or infection.

My experience (and that of many colleagues) is that parents who are sensitively informed of their child's situation are rarely rejecting— usually they are extremely supportive. Many patients will, of course, have grown away from their parents, perhaps having moved away from their home area in the first place because they could not tell them of their homosexuality. As time passes, the divide may seem to have grown greater, contributing to the patient's feeling that there would be no scope for understanding at all as a result. Other patients have expressed fears of the impact of their news on the health of elderly parents; they continue to 'hide' their situation from family members in order to avoid the possibility of hastening illness in their parents. Some may have argued with family members about their sexuality or lifestyles in the past, and choose to keep their news to themselves in order to avoid opening old emotional wounds on all sides. Yet, despite such approaches, I can think of only one or two families who have not responded to their child's news with great sadness and then firm emotional and/or practical support. It seems that the life experience and greater world-weary resilience in the perspectives of the older generation are often forgotten by younger persons, who probably remember only how their parents reacted to stresses when they were the patient's age. It is certainly interesting to me to observe that greater levels of deprecating moralising about AIDS and HIV come from patients than from their families, and their parents in particular, during the period immediately following diagnosis.

This does depend to some extent on the closeness of the family in the first place, and on the level of accurate information that they have about AIDS and HIV. The need to provide clear and understandable information to families is just as great as it is for other persons in the patient's life. This is particularly so in those instances where the family has been hitherto unaware of the patient's lifestyle, and news of the illness leads to a double awareness—of lifestyle and of disease. One father said it this way:

> I did not know that Philip was homosexual and feel very sorry that he felt he couldn't tell me. I don't like it, but I can get used to it. I think he was afraid that I would turn him out, especially now that he has got AIDS. However, he is my son and I love him, and that comes before anything else.

In some cases, parents and families have only been informed of the situation by patients in the terminal stages of illness, when the impact of the news is compounded by the grief of the parents, who have possibly not had sufficient time to adjust to the situation and to talk it through with their child. In other cases the illness may prompt a family reunion after years of separation caused by the pains of growing and 'coming out'. Frequently, hospital counsellors will provide a setting for 'family therapy' or discussion, so that issues related to the infection/ disease and their child's sexuality or lifestyle can be aired in the company of skilled and sensitive guides.

As suggested elsewhere in this book, one of the biggest difficulties for families and friends of people with HIV is to know how best to help. Some may 'overhelp' and thus either encourage patients to sit back and become passive or encourage them to see themselves as a sort of sick 'victim'. It is clearly important to avoid overhelping, but striking a useful medium can be tricky. The Gay Counselling Service of New South Wales, Australia, has produced some useful tips for those who are trying to find that medium between avoidance and overhelping.

1. When friends have AIDS or HIV, don't avoid them. Showing support by visiting helps to instil hope and motivation to carry on and fight. The temptation may be to change the way you speak to the patient, but talk to him or her the way you always have— familiarity and consistency are important for the patient's self-esteem.
2. Don't be afraid to touch the patient—a squeeze of the hand or a hug is a simple way of showing that you care.

3. Telephone before you visit, in case the patient is not feeling up to having visitors that day. And don't be put off if you are asked not to call that day—the patient may be lonely as well as ill.
4. Don't be afraid to show your emotions when the patient does—sharing tears can be as important as sharing laughs, and demonstrates to the patient that he or she is not alone.
5. Providing 'treats' can be a huge morale booster—e.g. bringing a favourite meal around or preparing one together; walking or visiting favourite places; bringing books, videos, tapes; or going to a party or a show together.
6. Include the patient in holiday and festival celebrations—bring cards, pictures, flowers, etc., to decorate the hospital room or home; organise phone calls, letters and visits from other friends, too.
7. Offer to help with any difficult correspondence or negotiations that may be troubling the patient.
8. Offer to help lovers/spouses/families as well, by giving them 'breaks' from the care of the patient, inviting them out, letting them talk, and so on.
9. If the patient has children, offer to take them out or to help care for them for a short while.
10. Don't be reluctant to ask about the patient's illness or infection—he or she may need to talk to someone (else) about it and how he or she is managing. Start by asking, 'Do you feel like talking about it?'
11. Don't feel that you both always have to talk—sitting together reading, listening to music or watching television can be restful and enriching. Words sometimes get in the way!
12. If you have a car, you may be able to help by transporting your friend to particular places, or by just taking him or her for a drive to 'get out of the house' or hospital for a while.
13. Encouragement is vital. If the patient is looking better, tell him or her so. If his or her appearance is changing for the worse, it may be useful to acknowledge the fact, but only if you can do so with sensitivity and gentleness. It is always important not to lie.
14. Keep involving the patient in decision-making; encourage him or her to feel that he or she still has control over his or her life, even if it is diminished by the process of illness and hospitalisation.
15. Tell the patient what you would like to do for him or her, and if he or she agrees, keep your promise to do it.
16. If the patient gets angry with you for no obvious reason, don't take it personally—remember that the patient is enduring tremendous frustration and fear, and that it is your very closeness that may make the demonstration of anger possible.

17. Most people like gossip—keep them informed of what's happening outside, with whom and when. Take your cues from the patient about topics of conversation. Discussing current events will help the patient to feel that the world is not 'passing them by'.
18. Offering to take care of household chores may bring enormous relief, especially if the patient has pets or plants that need attention while he or she is in hospital. But take care not to do things that the patient can do unaided (see above), and to ask before you do anything.
19. If you have a strong religious faith, and the patient does also, ask if you could pray for or with him or her. Patients may take comfort from your acceptance of their spiritual needs and practices, and from having passages from the Bible, Koran or other spiritual books read to them at times.
20. It is important to bring a positive attitude to your meetings with the patient, but be careful to take your cues from the patient and from your experience of his or her moods prior to the present illness or infection. Don't create a tyranny of positive thinking that can lead to feelings of guilt and blame for not getting better.
21. Have a sense of history about the patient's illness/infection and his or her reactions to it. There will be 'up days' and 'down days' which no amount of well-meaning chat can interrupt. Use these experiences to help both you and the patient develop a sense of perspective over the circumstances.
22. Do not confuse acceptance of the illness/infection with defeatism. Experience shows that acceptance is a positive step in developing a sense of mastery over the virus and its effects. In a similar vein, don't be afraid to talk about the future and the things that may happen (including the possible development of disease)—planning reinforces hope, provides a sense of perspective and helps to make fear manageable.

It is important to realise that the burden of illness will sometimes lead to the end of a friendship, and that this is as natural as the cementing of close friendships which can also occur. Some people cannot move at the same speed as the ill person, and become intolerant, for example, of the patient's reduced capacity for the previous lifestyle, of his or her 'AIDS evangelism', or of his or her sadness at the changed circumstances. Perhaps some friends become frightened or vulnerable if disease is discussed or becomes visible, or they simply don't know how to provide support. In some cases such partings may be more helpful to the patient than lingering awkwardness and tensions over the new circumstances.

PLANNING FOR BEREAVEMENT

> This is something I've had most problems with. My children, my friends and my family *will not* discuss it, and if I insist on doing so, I'm generally told that I'm being morbid and to shut up. They fail to grasp my situation.

Where loved ones are involved, the realisation that death may come is obviously painful and distressing, and it is natural that such discussion may be avoided or dismissed: everyone wants to hope for (and see) the best. The subject of bereavement and preparing for it is too large to be comprehensively dealt with in this book. Those wishing to read further about the processes of dying and bereavement are referred to *Facing Death: Patients, Families and Professionals*, by Averil Stedeford (Heinemann, London, 1984). However, it is important to recognise the significance of this issue for patients. It has already been stated that those who have the greatest capacity to live for and enjoy the present are those, generally, who have managed to accept their illness and the possibility of death. Therefore, it is important to assist that process of acceptance, usually by allowing patient discussion and the making of plans to help tie up 'loose ends'.

The psychological and psychosocial issues discussed elsewhere in this book are all closely bound up in the process of patient bereavement (for the life they may lose). Characteristically, the need to keep talking is most important to help the anxieties and concerns associated with death and dying bubble through to the surface—to help the patient sort his or her life and death out in his or her own mind. However, this is not always easy for the loved ones, particularly if the patient currently is well and responding to treatment. Talk of death may be interpreted quite wrongly as a depressive response to manageable circumstances, and be met with what seems to be a desperately cheerful avoidance of the facts. Within close relationships, there may be much less discussion of death, simply because mutual understanding surpasses the need for words. In other relationships, however, talking may have to be encouraged and, to some extent, organised so that important issues are actually brought out into the open. Again, rehearsing what you want to say, and how you say it, can be an important help. You can use a counsellor or friend to practise with before bringing the subject up 'cold' with a loved one.

Ill or dying patients are often placed in the role of main comforter to those whom they love and who love them. They may, after all, have a deeper, more direct acceptance of their own possible death than those who are placed in the role of most reluctant observers. This can lead to strains and ruptures within close relationships, particularly if the lover is unprepared to accept things the way the patient does. It seems unnatural and unfair to many patients that they have to look after their loved one when the loved one should really be looking after them. Further strains may appear in times of critical illness, when patients appear to turn to their parents, or to those whom they have known since they were small, for more support and sharing than to their lover or spouse. This occurs particularly in younger couples, perhaps where the bonds of the loving relationship are not as strong or secure as in the older, more established relationships.

Seriously ill people may show a wide range of reactions to their situation which complicate the process of coming to terms with declining health or death. We have already considered the effects of depression, anxiety and other psychological responses in earlier chapters. In addition, many patients in the terminal stages of AIDS may show signs of mental confusion, personality changes and other signs that often accompany neurological disease but also appear with no such apparent complications. Much of the distress created by such changes can be successfully treated by medication and good nursing management, but there will still be much distress for the lover/family of the dying patient. Perhaps a more universal feature of those who are seriously ill or dying is the feeling of guilt for leaving behind all their responsibilities and burdens, or for the pain they are causing their loved ones. In such cases, making appropriate plans together can help greatly to relieve the burden of guilt. This is how one member of the PWA Group put it:

> Making a will and tying-up loose ends was important, as it helped to relieve some stress about the mess one might leave behind for my family and lover.

It can be difficult to know when to bring such an issue up—one doesn't wish to encourage alarm or despondency in the patient who is otherwise feeling quite well and fit! However, it is appropriate to do so when the patient wishes, and to offer what legal and practical help one can, so that further uncertainties are diminished.

Perhaps it is important to emphasise that fear is almost always destructive, particularly of confidence. If you fear to be honest with your loved one about the future and his or her illness, he or she may lose confidence in your own ability to cope (just as you might). Making one's self vulnerable to discussion and rebuke is a way of making one's self stronger by facing up to the future and its potential. A sense of mastery and peace with one's self will only come if honesty and sensitivity prevail.

7

Summary and Reports from Veterans

Over the months of writing this book, one major change in the social approach to those with AIDS and HIV infection has occurred: a Government-sponsored education campaign has emphasised that AIDS is not a 'gay disease'. All sexually active persons with more than one partner are potentially at risk of exposure to this infection if they do not take personal responsibility for infection control and use condoms and lubricants. However, rather than providing a reassuring message for the general population, many have been frightened and new fuel has been added to the arguments of the 'moral right' in their denunciation of those persons most at risk of future infection and disease. So, despite the recent Government involvement, there is more than ever a need for sober and clear discussion of the facts of HIV and its (personal) management.

RELIGIOUS ISSUES

Many patients have been particularly disturbed by the religious emphasis brought out in discussion of AIDS and AIDS patients. Guilt is a very destructive feeling, and many people rightly feel that sections of society are blaming them for the fact of AIDS and HIV. Biblical authority is often invoked in the blaming process, particularly where homosexuality is being discussed. Because homosexuality is described as sinful in parts of the Bible, the advent of AIDS is held up as proof of 'God's wrath' and as a vindication of antihomosexual feeling.

I believe that it is a mistake to get heavily drawn into such lines of argument, mainly because they are bound never to be resolved. A stern reliance on written prose and ideology can rarely be overcome by rational counter-argument: the critic has already made his or her 'leap of faith', which, in zealots, determines that any attempt to argue against their convictions is sure evidence of the need for the moral change that they ardently seek. Such persons are not persuaded by facts, such as lesbians being the safest group for infection-free sexual contact; the evidence from Africa showing that 99 per cent of people with AIDS are in heterosexual groups (even after allowing for non-sexual transmission, the proportion of homosexuals in the total of people with AIDS is minuscule); or the fact that one need not be promiscuous in order to become infected—I have had a number of patients who became HIV seropositive after their first episode of sexual intercourse. To many people, biblical authority is itself suspect: who, these days, would agree with the book of Leviticus that any woman found guilty of adultery should be put to death (by being stoned within sight of the walls of her own village), or that any couple having sexual relations while the woman is menstruating should be cast out and shunned by society? These suggestions are found alongside that which says that homosexual men should be put to death.

Significantly, not all clergy are antigay or so ready and willing to denounce homosexuals for their association with AIDS. In fact, it seems likely that most do respond to the tragedy of AIDS with the kind of Christian compassion and concern that we would expect. For most people, AIDS is a reality that cannot be argued out of existence, just as we cannot argue people out of buying cars and killing themselves and others in car crashes. It is important to many people with AIDS and HIV to make peace with themselves and find spiritual acceptance as part of their response to infection and disease. That any people could wish to complicate such personal searches by immoderate and destructive interpretations of their own beliefs surely says more about the critic's blind dogma than the patient's individual needs.

SUMMING UP

This book is about managing a crucial, life-threatening infection and the disease states it can give rise to. It concerns the benefits of making an *active* response to this situation, rather than having a reliance on others or a helpless acceptance of the circumstances. It has always aimed at realism rather than false optimism, while also admitting room for *hope*.

A doctor friend who has been under intense pressure since working in the field was asked about how she coped with the present reality of so many AIDS deaths. She said:

> I do get depressed at times, but I have to tell myself that many patients are well, that many of the opportunistic infections we see can be successfully treated, and that one day—before too long—a cure will come.

Her honest expression is mirrored by the words of many others who are facing this disease far more directly. Charles, when asked to sum up his experiences, wrote:

> I often visualise the virus as an alien creature that has invaded my body. I talk to it, argue with it and curse it! I feel a battle of wills between me and IT and I'm determined to emerge the winner with it shrivelling up and dying.
>
> I go to great lengths to maintain my appearance, both by the clothes I wear, keeping fit and I hope good grooming. All this and inner strengths that I didn't know I had until AIDS have enabled me to maintain and even improve on my self-confidence. I am in control and proud of myself.
>
> Meeting other people with AIDS has been of great help, both in not feeling alone, being inspired by their positive attitudes and learning about other methods of coping. While appreciating my own enormous good fortune in many respects, especially in that I have never been ill, I hope that sometimes someone will get encouragement from my approach. Informal gatherings such as discos, etc., are a great help in bringing one back into the community after a period of isolation.

Peter, a person with HIV infection only, who has written a great deal about his trauma and adjustment, made his conclusion as follows:

> People in my position do not want pity. What we do want is for people to realise that we are not in the least dangerous to other people save for the most intimate sexual contact. We need the love and support of our friends and money to be spent on looking for a cure.

All of the people whose ideas and statements have contributed to this book have faced their infection and/or diseases as individuals. They have each made their own way through the dark passages of fear, depression, consuming worry, guilt and all the other issues that have been discussed. It is fair to say that, for most, these dark passages have led to new horizons of self-understanding. Learning to live with AIDS and HIV is often a process of self-discovery that can lead to an enrichment and acceptance that may never have been considered possible by those who have had the courage and determination to do so. There is no real correct way—each must find it for himself. It is the hope of all of us in the People with AIDS Group that this book will be helpful in guiding others along those twisting and challenging paths.

Perhaps, if nothing else, it does affirm the earlier suggestion that you are not alone.

To finish this book, Grahame, a founder member of the Group, has written a personal statement which explains his own life with AIDS. It is perhaps typical of the range of issues many others have faced.

Back in early September 1984 I was diagnosed as having Kaposi's Sarcoma and therefore AIDS.

I had noticed two small marks on one of my legs in February '84. Aware of my sexual contact with a guy who had developed AIDS, I went to my Sexually Transmitted Diseases clinic and explained the facts. It wasn't until 2nd September '84 that I had a biopsy on these lesions and Kaposi's Sarcoma (KS) was subsequently diagnosed.

Despite my having been convinced for several months that the marks were KS, it still came as a bombshell when the doctor gave me the diagnosis—it was as though someone had put my head on a block and chopped it off! The first contact I was aware of had died by this point. I have subsequently found that two of my other sexual partners also had AIDS.

So began a complete change in my lifestyle and, I'm glad to say, 18 months later, as far as the outside world would know, I'm still the same person, alive and well. However, with the realisation that I have what is generally known as a 'terminal illness', I decided from Day One that I wouldn't accept the finality of my diagnosis, but that I would survive.

The following weeks proved to be very important in formulating my lines of defence, and eventual attack on the virus. Fortunately, I had enjoyed reasonable health, being a fit and athletic guy and, up to the diagnosis, I hadn't had any of the symptoms often experienced by people who are HTLV III antibody positive. A year and a half have passed since diagnosis and I'm still in good health and, although I've had the odd cold and one or two minor problems, they're only what you would expect in everyday life.

One of the first things I did, on the advice of the doctor at the clinic, was to contact the Terry Higgins Trust and was told about the AIDS Support Group. I was also put in contact with a sympathetic doctor who became my GP—a very useful advisor to have.

The first few Support Group meetings I attended were of enormous psychological help to me—I was able to talk openly to guys in the same boat as me, receive encouragement, ask the dozens of questions that were going through my head, and get answers from people who had faced the same problems, such as family, friends, work, health, emotions and home life. I try never to miss a meeting. [They] seem to fly by—we have lots of laughs, but try to keep up to date with what's going on medical-wise, and offer support to those who need it. It is sad and depressing when you see friends deteriorate over a period of time, but one of the first things we agreed was that people should always be made welcome no matter how ill they look, and our sick friends should always feel there is a welcome for them at our meetings.

In October '84 I attended a workshop about 'Psychological Aspects of AIDS'. It summed up many of the changes that had happened to me since I began to fear the marks on my body were KS, and that had continued since diagnosis. These had manifested themselves in several ways, in my case, for example, in loss of self-esteem (the social leper syndrome) and fears of a change in my quality of life—social, occupational, physical, sexual and relationship fears. Anxiety and depression can have tremendous impact on the normal ways of coping with life. When I became aware that these reactions were normal under such circumstances, life was more tolerable—I realised I wasn't going mad!

At the time of my diagnosis I was beginning to supervise the refurbishment of a Georgian house I had bought a year previously and had been staying with a friend while waiting planning permission to commence work on the house. Looking back in my diary, I see an odd mixture of entries around that period. The day of my biopsy it read—'bought bathroom suite; hospital for biopsy on marks; met electrician and builder for site meeting'. A few days later I had to go to the STD clinic for minor treatment to another problem I had. The entry reads—'went to clinic for treatment; doctor gave me diagnosis of biopsy; home like a zombie; Bob (my other half with whom I was staying) invited friends for impromptu dinner party'. Those lines were very few and to the point. No words could have conveyed the way I felt, especially when I had to tell Bob the news in the ten minutes before the visitors arrived. Needless to say we weren't our usual selves that evening.

Bob and I had had an argument the week before and had been sleeping in separate rooms for a few nights. That night, more than any other in my life, I needed someone special to hold me very tight and care for me. I stayed alone, as much through my own stubborn choice as anything, cried a little but was in too much of a state of shock to have a good weep or to sleep. My news finished our relationship—perhaps we could have got back together under 'normal' circumstances. In the following months before I moved into my own house, we would sit at opposite ends of the sofa, just good friends.

Several months later I stayed in Holland with a former lover and I got my cuddle and feelings from someone I still felt deeply for—my tears flowed for the first time and I felt as though someone really cared.

Since those initial days I have told many of my friends my situation, and I'm sure the news has got around to others I know. Genuine support and concern from the vast majority of people has been considerable and much appreciated.

As a direct result of groundless fears I was sent home from work in January [1985] after news of my illness was given to colleagues. The timing of the disclosure to them came as the media 'launched' into its mass coverage of AIDS for the first time and consequently frightened certain of the people I worked with, and their families. Although I was medically fit for work, and still am, I have not been allowed back to work and am now on a permanent sickness insurance scheme. However, some of my strongest support and friendship comes from former work colleagues.

Having managed to keep my elderly mother in the dark about my illness and not being at work till quite recently, I now have to adjust to the realisation that she knows the full situation. As she lives alone, a long way from me, and is in bad health, I attempted to save her the anguish she is undoubtedly going through now for as long as possible. She has taken the news remarkably well, at least as well as I can see, and is 100 per cent supportive of the course of complementary treatment, spiritual healing and self-help I have decided to take. Although we have always been close, this has brought us even closer together. There is now no need for me to hide the facts from her as I had been doing. The acceptance of my situation, open talk about it and the genuine care of loved ones is of immense importance and comfort to me, and now I know I have that from all around me.

Grahame, May 1986

Subject Index